THE COMPLEAT ACADEMIC:

A Practical Guide for the Beginning Social Scientist

Edited by

Mark P. Zanna
University of Waterloo

and

John M. Darley
Princeton University

Sponsored by
the Society for the Psychological Study of Social Issues

RANDOM HOUSE

New York

Distributed by
Lawrence Erlbaum Associates, Publishers
Hillsdale, New Jersey, and London

First Edition
9 8 7 6 5 4 3

Published in the United States by Random House, Inc., and simultaneously in Canada by Random House of Canada Limited, Toronto.

Library of Congress Cataloging-in-Publication Data
The Compleat academic.
Bibliography: p.
1. Social sciences—Study and teaching.
2. Social sciences—Vocational guidance.
3. College teaching. I. Zanna, Mark P.
II. Darley, John M.
H62.C584825 1986 300'.7 86-17797
ISBN 0-394-35252-1 (paperback)
ISBN 0-394-37386-3 (hardcover)

Manufactured in the United States of America

To Chuck Kiesler and Elliot Aronson, each a Compleat Academic in his own right, who imparted to us informally as graduate students much of what we hope is conveyed herein in print.

CONTENTS

FOREWORD

It is my honor, as incumbent SPSSI president, to write a foreword to a book that I think will be truly unique in our field. This book, *The Compleat Academic: A Practical Guide for the Beginning Social Scientist,* has been very long in development, and has benefited from the support and effort of a number of SPSSI past presidents, publication chairs, and editorial advisors, in addition to its editors, Zanna and Darley, and the other eight contributors. Now, at last, the book is completed. And in my judgment, the product is well worth the effort and the wait.

The Compleat Academic is a compendium of information about a host of problems and concerns that beset the work and life of the beginning academic social scientist. It covers the period from the start of the senior graduate student's job search, through the new assistant professor's first years of research, teaching, and graduate student supervision. (There is also one chapter on a parallel portion of the life of the young social scientist who chooses to follow a non-academic career path.)

It is a veritable gold mine of information for young social science professionals who are in or plan to enter academic settings. Its topics range widely. It includes detailed recommendations about preparing and giving a job talk, discussion of hidden problems and opportunities involved in planning and organizing one's research projects in the new job setting, advice for avoiding a series of potential professional traps that can stunt or destroy a young academic career, tips on teaching and on writing, advice about scheduling and managing time on and off the job, and a discussion of the difficulties involved in adjusting to one's new role in the faculty–graduate student relation.

As I read the manuscript to prepare this foreword, I began by skimming rapidly to get the chore done, expecting to be bored by such mundane "professional" (as opposed to "intellectual") matters. I soon was thoroughly fascinated with the material, reading all the chapters I had at hand carefully and intensely. I found myself muttering: "Yes, that certainly happens to a lot of assistant professors;" "Very good, I never looked at it that way;" and "Great! New faculty need to know that and no one ever tells them." I found the material so compelling that I began making plans to get my preprint copies into the hands of my own graduate students before they went off on any more job interviews or new jobs.

The book deals with many troublesome issues that are recurrent themes in the experience of junior faculty members. It discusses issues such as:

What to do about opportunities to collaborate with a very senior colleague.
How to prevent getting involved in directing too many theses on topics that are not in your own areas of expertise.
How to prepare for, carry out, and improve lectures and other teaching activities.
How to plan time and stick to those time plans.
How to get the writing flowing when it stops, and how to get it properly channeled once it flows.

The book deals with these issues *from the point of view of the young faculty member's own experience,* and offers practical advice for handling them. The advice is pragmatic without being cynical. Most of the chapters deliberately propose solutions that are advantageous from the point of view of the young professional, without being Machiavellian in relation to the academic systems within which that assistant professor is working.

The problems raised are truly endemic to the academic. Remarkably, there is not a single problem raised in the chapters that I read that I have not personally seen lived out by colleagues, students, or myself. And the advice given in this book would have been valuable to the parties in a very large majority of those cases. Even in those instances in which the book's advice did not match my own preferred way of coping with a set of issues, the advice still did represent a sensible point of view that was apt to be effective for many junior faculty.

The book is aimed at young social science professionals, mainly those in academic settings. It is therefore also invaluable to the graduate student in anticipation of that set of roles. It may not seem on the face of it to be of much use to those of us who are already established in academic careers. But if my own experience is any guide it will turn out to be fascinating and useful, most of all, to those very people. After all, it is those now-established academics who will readily recognize the pervasiveness of the problems and the impact they can have. And it is those now established academics who will transmit our social science academic culture—with appropriate changes it is to be hoped—to future generations of researcher-teacher-scholars.

In my judgment, many of these issues need such self-conscious treatment in our graduate training. I am already making plans to use this book as the core text for a "professional problems" graduate seminar. I'll bet a lot of other people will do that too. I am pleased the SPSSI has played a useful role in bringing this valuable resource book to present and future members of our field.

J. E. McGrath
Urbana, Illinois

FOREWORD

As the chairperson of the Education and Training Board of the American Psychological Association, I am pleased to contribute this Foreword. I do not think there is a higher calling than to be a professor. But being a successful one does involve more than good intent, sound values, and a humanistic commitment. Hence, I resonate to this volume, *The Compleat Academic,* and I am also amused at the coincidence of the title. While in my first teaching position, I not only began to learn how to be a faculty member, but also learned the joys of fishing under the tutelage of the college's treasurer (a person who must surely have read the classic volume on fishing, *The Compleat Angler*).

In looking at the contents of this volume, I am aware of how "complete" it is and of how far we've come from that earlier book for academics, *The Academic Marketplace*. *The Compleat Academic* covers the structural issues of hiring, of developing a career, and of academic politics. It also gives advice useful for various academic tasks, including classroom teaching, research, scholarly activity and grantsmanship. Here the aspiring graduate student, the graduate on the market and the junior faculty member can discover the "rules of the game." In sum, *The Compleat Academic* should ensure that academia will have successful and talented faculty, and that gifted faculty will be able to fully develop their talents. Ultimately, the institution, the faculty member, and the student benefit . . . and this is what education and training is all about.

Richard M. Suinn, Chairperson
Education & Training Board
American Psychological Association
Professor of Psychology & Head
Department of Psychology
Colorado State University

PREFACE

It is now customary to analyze any complicated corner of society as a "game." This metaphor implies that there are clear rules, known to all, and that, as a consequence, those who win the game are those who have the most skills and talents. An alternative explanation is possible, however: understanding the "rules of the game" gives the advantage. Thus those for whom the rules have never been spelled out may well achieve less than those with more savvy. More importantly, they may well achieve less than their talents might have led them to do had they been more thoroughly schooled in the rules.

It strikes us that this latter case is often true for those playing the "academic game." A number of people have less success than they might, not because they have fewer talents, but because they do not have a complete understanding of the "system" within which they are working. If this is true, then we are wasting a great many talents within academe. The teaching, the research, and the scholarship done in the academic setting is of such vital importance that any loss of talent seems to us to be a tragedy. There is also a moral issue; if some individuals succeed because they understand the rules of the game, while others fail because they do not, then a basic unfairness has been perpetrated.

Our own consideration of the implicit rules of the academic enterprize led to the development of the present book. In it a number of experienced academics attempt to convey "the rules of the academic game" to prospective faculty members. We attempt to shed light on some of the complex issues to be faced by individuals contemplating making their way in academic and research professions. Hitherto, we argue, most of this information has been learned by trial and error or selectively passed on orally. It certainly has not been communicated explicitly or systematically to senior graduate students and beginning faculty members. While we by no means claim that this volume says all that needs to be said, we have begun the task of making some of these considerations both explicit and public.

This book is published under the auspices of The Society for the Psychological Study of Social Issues, an organization with a long and honorable tradition of societal concern. This means that a vast majority of the authors are themselves psychologists and, therefore, many of the examples on which they draw are taken from psychology. However, we believe the book is relevant to a wider audience. The reactions of individuals to whom we have shown various of the chapters suggest that the book has broad applicability within psychology. We suspect it has applicability within the social sciences, and possibly, within the humanities and physical sciences as well. Therefore, our target audience is the senior graduate student or beginning faculty member at an institution that values both teaching and good research. We also have something to say to the increasing number of social scientists who are contemplating non-academic research careers.

In demonstrating the utility of a particular approach, it is always useful to point out specific examples. In demonstrating the utility of this sort of book, time and again we found it useful to point to concrete examples of materials written to advise our target audience. More often than not, these materials had been written by Daryl Bem and Bill McKeachie. We are particularly pleased that the work of each is represented within this volume. We are pleased as well by the enthusiastic response of our other authors who have been willing to take the time and trouble to summarize what they have learned and communicate it with grace and enthusiasm to others. It is a pleasure to express our own gratitude, and that of The Society for the Psychological Study of Social Issues, to the chapter authors of this volume.

Finally, like many volunteer efforts, this book has a lengthy prepublication history. It was continuously supported throughout these times by several SPSSI publication representatives, including Marilynn Brewer, Dan Perlman, Jeff Rubin, Reuben Baron, and Louise Kidder.

Preparation of this work has been substantially aided as well by the University of Waterloo and Princeton University, both of which provided facilities and resources, including sabbatical leaves. The editors' last efforts on the book were accomplished during a year that John Darley spent as a Fellow at the Center for Advanced Studies in the Behavioral Sciences, and he is grateful for the financial support provided by the National Science Foundation, #BNS-8011494, and by the John D. & Catherine T. MacArthur Foundation.

This book says something, but not everything, about a number of problems a beginning academic will face. While some of what is said may be wrong, it is more likely that many more things will need to be qualified in terms of the context in which the reader finds him- or herself. It would be a mistake to consider this book the definitive source. Rather, we hope that it will initiate discussion among faculty, and faculty and graduate students about the topics on which we touch. Further, we would hope that issues of "professionalism" and academic pitfalls would become legitimate topics of discussion, and even the focus of graduate seminars.

The Society for the Psychological Study of Social Issues has been encouraging about the possibility of a second edition. If this proves to be the case, it will be vital for us to have comments and suggestions from readers of the volume. For that reason, we encourage you to write either of us. We would be interested in hearing from readers about which concerns we have covered insufficiently or inaccurately. We also suspect that there are important topics on which we have not touched, and we ought to hear about those as well. It would also be helpful, for future editions, and perhaps the contributors' egos, to hear about sections that strike the reader as particularly accurate or useful.

Finally, we would like to invite you to tell us about your favorite article (published or unpublished) on any professional issue so that we can begin to develop a "compleat" list of Recommended Readings for the next edition. To start this list each of us has submitted a favorite article. Our two nominees appear in the Appendix of this volume.

Mark P. Zanna
Department of Psychology
University of Waterloo
Waterloo, Ontario N2L 3G1
Canada

John M. Darley
Department of Psychology
Princeton University
Princeton, New Jersey 08544
U.S.A.

I GETTING AND STARTING AN ASSISTANT PROFESSORSHIP

1
THE HIRING PROCESS IN ACADEMIA

John M. Darley
Princeton University

Mark P. Zanna
University of Waterloo

As faculty members whose university careers have spanned more years and more colleges than we care to remember, we have frequently been involved in the process of hiring new faculty members. One overwhelming discrepancy about the process strikes us: University and college departments of psychology have a set of procedures and rules by which they hire new faculty members, but these rules are rarely known or understood by the job applicants. As a result, we have seen excellent graduate students present themselves poorly and fail to get good jobs. Your task during the hiring process is to put yourself forward as an autonomous, self-organized, and self-starting individual; hopefully, this chapter will help you to do so.

THE BEGINNING: IDENTIFYING AND APPLYING FOR POSSIBLE JOBS

Your Faculty References

In the fall of your last year of graduate school, decide which three or four faculty know the most about you. In addition to your research advisor, consider faculty with whom you have done research or taught, or from whom you have taken sufficient course work so that they can give a confident estimate of the range of your skills and talents.

Next comes an extremely important step: discuss with your advisor the kind of job for which you are looking. What sort of balance of teaching, research, and practice are you seeking? Is your research likely to be basic or applied? Do you seek a college, university, or applied setting? Remind your advisor of those experiences that qualify you for various jobs so that they can be commented on in your advisor's letter. Also, find out the faculty's perception of your skills and talents; their verbal and written recommendations will be critical in determining your job possibilities. Out of this discussion will emerge some kind of definition of the appropriate job for you to seek.

Finding Possible Jobs

Scan the *APA Monitor,* the *CPA Highlights,* the *Chronicle of Higher Education,* and the newsletters and publications of various APA and CPA divisions and interest groups. Also, faculty members at your university may receive letters asking them for nominations for jobs. If these letters are kept in a central file, look through it; faculty members often receive these announcements prior to their publication in official bulletins.

As you are no doubt aware, the current job market is tight. Consequently, you are not likely to find or get your "perfect" job; this fact will affect your job search in various ways. First, although this article is mainly about getting an academic job in psychology, because that's what we know about, you should definitely explore non-academic job possibilities. Industry, the federal and state/provincial governments, and school systems all employ psychologists. A number of excellent articles about these sorts of jobs can be found in Woods' (1976) *Career Opportunities for Psychologists* (see also DeJong & Saxe, this volume). Talk to faculty members about these other job possibilities, but remember that they may not have as complete a network of contacts outside the academic community as they have within it. If any recent graduates from your Ph.D. program have taken industrial or government jobs, learn what you can from them. If there is a business or medical school at your institution, talk to any psychologists working there and find out what they do and how they got their jobs.

Another job possibility is the 1- or 2-year postdoctoral position. It gives you a chance to do research relatively free from the teaching pressures of a normal beginning faculty job (although getting some teaching experience while on a postdoctoral fellowship is advisable). Primarily for this reason, postdoctoral fellowships may be an increasingly desirable alternative in all fields of psychology. Sources of money for postdoctoral work seem to be expanding in Canada (e.g., Social Sciences and Humanities Research Council, Natural Sciences and Engineering Research Council) and, if not expanding in the United States, at least not contracting, so do seek out information about such opportunities.

When exploring any or all of these alternatives, don't let geographic or lifestyle preferences rule out otherwise excellent jobs. Some about-to-be Ph.D's decide they have always wanted to live in a warm and benign climate and wish to limit their job search to California or British Columbia (Lemmings). Others feel that it would be impossible for them to live outside large urban environments (City Slickers). Still others feel they could not survive within those confines (Back to Nature). It is perfectly reasonable to hope that you will get a good job in one of your favorite places, but it is totally unreasonable to refuse to look at jobs that don't match these preferences. Your lifestyle is important to you, but so is your career.

One very real limit to job search flexibility is imposed by spouse career commitments. Many married couples deal with this problem, at least for a year or so, by living geographically separated, but we also know a lot of divorces that have resulted from this sort of pressure. Articles in the *American Psychologist* (e.g., Bryson, Bryson, Licht, & Licht, 1976; Madell & Madell, 1979; Matthews & Matthews, 1978) have presented several points of view on the problems of professional pairs that might be of interest to you.

If your search is restricted, consider writing a blanket letter to all the institutions that are possible for you, even if they have not advertised a vacancy. They may discover one when the fall teaching term begins. (See Grinder, 1976, for a more extended discussion of the use of unsolicited letters.)

Another potential job search restriction is imposed by the American/Canadian border. On the basis of his experience, Iacono (1981) argues that it is easier for Americans to obtain jobs at Canadian universities than vice versa, because American universities will only bother with immigration procedure hassles for outstanding foreign candidates. We have the feeling that the situation varies considerably depending on both the candidate and the institution; on balance, we would suggest that you apply for every job in which you are interested regardless of which side of the border it's on.

One final note: Don't apply for a job outside a geographical area if, when you stop to consider it, you know you wouldn't take it. It is insulting to the institution that offers you the job, creates bad will for your advisor, and blocks the offering of the job to candidates who really want it.

The Vita

Your vita is a very important document. With your reference letters, it determines the jobs for which you will be considered. There is no single, set format for the vita; start by listing everything you have done and then review your vita to make sure that it displays *all* your relevant skills (e.g., if you have been a Teaching Assistant, remember to include a summary of your teacher evaluations), interests, and talents. If some of these skills are not obviously documented, include paragraphs describing them. Also include paragraphs indicating your work "in progress," especially your thesis proposal, and your future research directions. Read the paper on vita preparation by Crossman and Nazzaro (1976), and look at the vitae prepared by graduate students senior to you. Treat your vita as you would any other manuscript. Present your first draft to several faculty members, including your advisor, for comments and revise.

You might also include a list of courses you could teach. Be neither parochial nor grandiose; do not suggest five courses that on examination prove to be variants on your thesis, but, on the other hand, don't claim to be able to teach every conceivable course in the university catalogue. Psychology departments are frequently looking for introductory psychology and statistics course teachers. If you are capable of teaching such courses and interested in doing so, say so on your vita. However, this claim is to be regarded as a commitment. Don't make it lightly.

Your papers and publications will be a major element of your vita and a frequent question is whether to send them. We think you should. Reprints are not bulky and are useful to committees making decisions about whom to invite. Also send papers given at conventions and reprints of papers in press. Don't send papers in preparation or under editorial review unless you are convinced that the write-up adequately presents the research. First drafts rarely do so.

Getting the Complete Record to the Hiring Institution

When hiring institutions are ready to make their decisions, they will choose from among those candidates with complete files. Make sure that you are one of them. Job advertisements often include application deadlines implying that you have several months to complete your file. Don't wait! Do not allow yourself to be seduced by fantasies about how much more impressive your vita will be tomorrow when you write up that old data, or when your three convention presentations are accepted, or when that journal editor finally gets around to making a decision on your manuscript. Some institutions will begin narrowing the field and issuing invitations long before the advertised deadline, so get your materials in early. (You can always send an "addendum" to your vita at a later point in time.)

A complete job application typically consists of your vita, whatever reprints you think are appropriate, a letter from your advisor and two other faculty members, and perhaps, but not necessarily, a letter from you. Give your letter writers the necessary addresses and tactfully check back with them after a decent interval to see that they have actually mailed the letters. The faculty recognize that these letters are critical to your career, but they are busy people and this kind of letter is difficult to write. Therefore they need a good deal of lead time, especially for the first letter requested.

The Hiring System (Such As It Is)

Having sent off all your materials, you must now endure the discomfort of waiting for a reply. The wait may be a long one and the response, when it comes, may not be what you were expecting, so be prepared! The academic hiring system is not a model of efficiency. The people making the hiring decisions are faculty members who have backed into taking that responsibility. They are overloaded, they are not professionals at hiring, and they tend not to be completely organized. They are also probably somewhat embarrassed at having such great decision-making power over other people's lives. As a result, the communications you do receive may be somewhat unclear or even, if coming from several sources, apparently contradictory. (Greaves' 1979 guide to securing a position in psychology is an excellent source of information about the motivations of those doing the hiring; it also includes more extensive discussions of vita preparation and other topics mentioned briefly here.)

Obviously, the high ambiguity of the hiring situation will make you anxious and/or depressed. If you are not invited for an interview, you will feel anger at the people there and suspicion that your faculty reference writers are not pushing you hard enough. Simultaneously, you will feel despair about your own skills, abilities, and self-worth. Expect all this; it is easier if you are prepared for it.

BEFORE YOUR VISIT

Let us assume that the happy event has occurred and you have been invited for a job visit. Congratulations! You have already achieved a great deal. Universities receive hundreds of applications for every position they advertise, and typically don't invite more than three or four people for an interview. Jobs are scarce and to be considered for one is no mean feat. Let us now tell you some things that will increase your chances of getting the job.

1. Set up your travel plans in advance. Before you respond to the invitation, check your schedule and travel arrangements. When could you visit? How can you get there? The only items of travel information you

should expect your contact person to provide are local transportation details and accommodation arrangements. This is your first chance to present yourself as an organized and effective individual. Don't miss it.

2. Research the institution before you visit it. Read the catalogues on file at your university for background information. Is it rural or urban? What is its history? What are its strengths and sources of pride? Seek out the faculty members in your psychology department who know something about the institution and learn about it from them.

3. Research the department you will be visiting. When invited to give a talk, you might ask your contact person to send you the brochure(s) the department has prepared for prospective graduate students, or simply get the faculty list from the most recent university catalogue and then, for people outside your own research area, learn in general what they do. For the people near your own area, review what they have published. Look for some of their work in the *Psychological Abstracts*. Read some of it. And, particularly if there are some individuals whose work is close to your own, know it very well.

4. Find out before (or during the visit) as much as you can about the search process. Although we know of only two case studies of this process (Quereshi, 1980, 1983), you should be able to find informants who can answer questions about the search procedure of the institution you are visiting. Are several candidates usually interviewed or only a few? Do faculty members get to vote on job candidates or are hiring decisions made solely by the search committee and/or department chairperson? Regarding the job you are applying for, is the department looking for an excellent general candidate or are skills specific to a particular area more important?

5. Find out about the talk. Most hiring institutions expect a candidate to give a talk, but *not* all hiring institutions convey these expectations clearly; some use quaint code words such as "say a few words to a few of us about your research." When you respond to the invitation, find out *exactly* what sort of talk is expected. At this time, you could also mention the kind of equipment you will need for your talk as well as its title.

THE TALK THAT GETS OR LOSES THE JOB

Its Importance. For better or worse, your talk may be the single most important determinant of whether you get the job offer. The way in which you present your material is thought to tell a great deal about your research and teaching abilities, your ability to think on your feet, and your overall personal style. For many of the faculty, your talk is the only contact they will have with you, and so their impressions will be formed considerably by it. When preparing and practicing the talk, think of it as a performance, and remember that a performance works best when it has been carefully scripted and when the performer has total control of the material. (A good discussion of this perspective is found in Perlman and Perlman's 1981 article on giving successful convention papers.)

What to Talk About. A talk goes better if it is on completed research; a feeling of anti-climax is inevitable if hypotheses are proposed and a method laid out, but no data can be presented. On the other hand, if you propose to follow your thesis up in future research, then you should talk about it, even if you do not have data. Your thesis also presumably reflects more of your own thinking than other research you may have done with your advisor so presentation of your thesis may help to establish the independence of your work from that of your advisor. Ideally, you have at least some data and can tell a story in progress, bringing people along with you through the chapters. This approach can make for an extraordinarily exciting colloquium.

Who Will be in the Audience? The key audience will be faculty members and perhaps advanced graduate students. If the institution does not have a graduate program, undergraduate students will be an important segment of the audience. Psychologists from every area are often involved in the decision-making progress and are likely to attend your talk. The mixed nature of your audience means that although you can assume that everybody is familiar with general psychological language, you should explain more specialized terms. You also need to explain your research context in enough detail so that audience members outside your own research field can understand it. A frequent after-colloquium comment is, "It was technically OK, but why did she want to do it in the first place?"

Length and Structure of the Talk. Your talk should be approximately 45 minutes long, fitting into a normal class hour and somewhat shorter than a regular colloquium. Present your ideas in a less complex way than you would in a written paper; oral comprehension is significantly poorer than reading comprehension.

Begin with an introduction that puts the work in a context understandable to psychologists in general and by implication makes clear the importance of the research. Refer to the historical background of your work and describe recent developments in the area, but do so succinctly. (Be sure to cite the individual who began the general research area and any researcher present at the talk!) After 10 minutes, you should have finished the introduction and be talking about your own work.

Unless your most important research innovation is procedural, present just enough procedural detail in your method section so that the audience is clear about what happened to the subjects. Mingle results and discussion sections, presenting a relatively small block of research and commenting on its meaning before moving on to the next block. For instance, you might first present the results that make clear that your manipulations worked and come to that conclusion; then go on to the results that speak to your hypothesis.

To end your talk, you could summarize what you have shown and make a brief but explicit statement regarding future research directions. Make very clear that you know the limits to what you have shown. All research has limits. People will be more impressed if you show a mature awareness that they exist.

Preparing Talk Details. If possible, use slides in your presentation, including pictures of apparatus, stimulus materials, and typical subjects in action. When presenting the research, you can lay out your design on a first slide, fill in control group results on a second slide, and then move to a third slide that includes the data from the experimental groups bearing on your hypothesis. With this approach, you can build your own suspense.

Make sure that both tables and figures are prepared and photographed so that they can be seen from a reasonable distance! Eliminate the last digits of your results rather than have them unreadable; it is the trend of the results that is important, not the exact numbers.

Alternatives to slides are writing the data on the blackboard as you talk or handing the data out beforehand in ditto form. People are likely to read a dittoed handout at inappropriate times. With blackboard data, you can control the rate at which it is presented, but it may be difficult for people to read, and may give a slightly amateur tone to your presentation. A reasonable compromise combines slides with a blackboard presentation of "hot off the press" data.

Practicing the Talk. Practice your colloquium not once but several times, taperecording or even videotaping your first attempt. Try it out on fellow graduate students, and then on faculty members, particularly those in other areas. Note what questions people ask, and begin to build some of the answers into the talk. You may not deal explicitly with all the questions that arise, but having heard them during the "rehearsal," you will be ready to answer them at the actual performance.

To Read or Not to Read the Talk. Knowing that they will be anxious initially and that it is important to set the context of the talk correctly, many people have the first few paragraphs of their talk written out in full. They also may have the last few paragraphs of the talk written so that they can state their conclusions precisely. In between, they rely on an outline and/or a series of slides to cue them. Other people are able to give a successful talk from a series of notes written on one sheet of paper or even with no notes at all. Past experience suggests to us that job candidates are not among those people.

WHAT YOU WANT TO KNOW ABOUT THE PLACE WHERE YOU MIGHT WORK

Information About the Department

Although you need the answers to quite a few questions, don't ask every question explicitly. During your visit, answers will frequently come unobtrusively and much of the necessary information will be volunteered. At some point, get off in a corner by yourself and look over your list of questions to see what answers you have. Determine what else you need to know and then tactfully ask about it.

1. What is the teaching load? How is it distributed between graduate and undergraduate courses? Are you needed for specific courses? Can you teach a new course? What are the typical class sizes? Is there a reduced teaching load for first-year faculty members? At American universities, can one obtain a "summer salary" by teaching in the summer term?
2. What sorts of teaching supports are available? Is there a well-stocked library with an organized reserve system? Is there a budget for xeroxing? For films? Are there graduate student teaching and/or research assistants? What norms govern teaching at the institution?
3. What are the department's expectations for faculty research? Does the department expect you to obtain a reseach grant and, if so, when? Some departments are structured so that departmental members rarely publish. Others expect a continuing stream of research output.
4. What space is available for your research? Would the space be yours alone or shared with other people? What are the sharing rules? Is space relatively plentiful or in short supply?
5. What sorts of support and equipment are available for your research? What about shop and computer facilities—what are they like and how are they billed? Does the institution allot "starter money" to

beginning faculty members for their research? Is money available for space modifications? Are travel funds available and, if so, what are the requirements for obtaining them? Is there a secretarial pool? Is it free or is it billed? What is its quality? (This is one area in which you can get faculty to talk freely and endlessly.)

6. How are research subjects obtained? Are there subject pools? Has contact been made with various school settings? How are infra-human subjects obtained? What are the animal care facilities? Are animal caretakers available or do you need to build up this sort of staff? Who pays?

7. What are the odds on getting promoted? What criteria do the department use for promotion? How are these decisions made? When? Historically, what has been the promotion rate? What is the possibility of getting tenure? Is the job, in fact, a "tenure stream" position? If not, what is the probability that it could become one? Find out whether budget or enrollment projections exist for the institution as a whole and the psychology department in particular and check them out. Such figures will provide some indication of the tenure situation. How does the situation "feel" to the junior faculty? Are they anxious and concerned about tenure and promotions? Is the possibility of collaboration reduced because they regard themselves as being in competition with one another? Is there a sharp division between the junior and senior faculty?

8. What is the consulting policy within the university? What is the pattern of consulting within the department?

9. What is the quality of the undergraduate students? (This question is especially important at a solely undergraduate institution.) In at least the advanced undergraduate courses, are they bright and well-motivated? What is the reputation of psychology as a major? What sort of expectations do the undergraduates have for contact with faculty members? Is there such a thing as an honors thesis? Who does it? Have any theses been published lately?

10. If the hiring institution has a graduate department, much of your research life will be spent with graduate students. Are they intelligent and motivated to do research? Do they help and support each other? Is there an active graduate student culture? What are their career aspirations? Historically, what sorts of placements have they received in the last few years? In what ways do they get involved in research? How are they supported? Do they have to spend unproductive time earning money to continue their graduate training? Are they full-time or part-time students? At some institutions, new faculty cannot supervise graduate students. If this is the case here, ask junior faculty what arrangements they make for conducting their research.

Information About the University

Because much of this information is standard, universities frequently have booklets that include it, particularly the less controversial elements.

1. What is the beginning salary? What has been the pattern of increases over the past few years? How were the increases determined?
2. What is the standard initial contract period? What is the standard renewal contract period?
3. Does the university provide moving expenses?
4. What is the sabbatical and leave of absence policy? It sometimes differs for junior and senior faculty. Make sure you understand it.
5. What are the university's retirement policies and what other benefits does it offer its faculty? Some universities have group health and/or life insurance plans, faculty medical and dental clinics, day care centers, and the like.
6. Every university has dimensions along which departmental contributions to the university are assessed. Determine the reward contingencies at this university. Is the department "paid off" for high national visibility of its faculty? Is its teaching efficiency important to the university administration? How is teaching efficiency measured?

In learning about a new department and university keep an open mind. We have often encountered candidates whom we would label "almamater"-centric. That is, they tend to assume that our university operates just like theirs and, worse, they are offended to discover that this isn't true, even when the differences involve rather trivial bureaucratic details. Our simple advice is don't assume every university is exactly alike!

Information About the Community

Although as a junior faculty member, you will undoubtedly be spending most of your time at the university, you *will* need somewhere to live! Find out the living circumstances of the other junior faculty. Does the university offer any assistance in finding and/or financing housing? Stop in at a local real estate agent and get some feel for area rents and costs. Pick up a local newspaper and check on houses for sale and apartments for rent.

Find out what employment opportunities exist for your spouse. The department you are visiting may not be set up to answer these questions but someone should be able to refer you to appropriate resource people. You should also check the general availability of day care centers and the quality of the schools your children would be attending.

Find out as much as you can about the physical, cultural, and recreational "climate" of the community. Will you have to buy an entirely new wardrobe and develop a taste for country music? What are the shopping facilities and restaurants like? These issues may not be critical in determining whether you take the job but they are important.

THINGS PEOPLE WILL WANT TO KNOW ABOUT YOU

Your "Classification." Faculty members, particularly those outside your own research area, will attempt to determine "the general context" of your psychological thinking. Within what research tradition are you working? Have you been affected by recent developments in psycholinguistics? Within social psychology, are you a cognitive social psychologist? You can describe yourself in a detailed way with faculty members in your own research area. But, when questioned by other faculty members, you should be prepared to place yourself reasonably accurately within psychology in one or two well-chosen sentences.

"The 5-Minute Drill." It is useful to be able to give one other sort of presentation. We have labeled it the "5-minute drill." Perhaps one faculty member missed your job talk; perhaps for another you want to describe a line (or future line) of research you didn't cover in your colloquium. We suggest that you be prepared to relate the theoretical context of your research, the specific hypotheses you are testing, the general procedures you are using to test them, and the outlines of the results you are getting (or would hope to get)—all in 5 minutes! Your major task is to convey the importance and excitement of this research succinctly so that you can, then, discuss your work with the person rather than lecture him or her during your time together.

To convey what you are up to without going into excessive detail is a surprisingly difficult task, and, at first, requires considerable thought and discipline. We suggest that you explicitly think through what you would say and practice it. When practicing, keep in mind that you may be relating your research to a colleague in another area who may need to know a bit more about some aspect (e.g., methods) of the research. Our advice is think through, in advance, modifications of your presentation as a function of a variety of possible audiences.

Although we believe the ability to present your research in capsule form will be useful on job interviews, we also want to point out that this form of presentation is, in fact, the way experienced psychologists communicate with one another about their research at conventions, conferences, or on colloquium visits. To be able to do this well indicates not only that you communicate effectively about your research, but also that you are able to demonstrate that there is one more way in which you fit the prototype of the effective psychologist.

Teaching. Think about what you want to teach. For those courses you want to teach and for those you will be expected to teach, have some ideas about what texts you will use and the general nature of the topics you would cover. Evidence that you have investigated the department's teaching needs and patterns shows your organization and your interest in the institution and suggests that you will be a good teacher.

Hidden Agendas. Inevitably, there will be some reservations concerning the merits of your candidacy. Typically, these reservations originate from two sources. First, concerns arise from a department's multiple needs, or from faculty members' various perceptions of the needs of the department. For example, the undergraduate advisor may have been counting on you to teach introductory psychology. Someone else may have been planning on getting someone to help out with the undergraduate and/or graduate courses in statistics. Still others may have hoped that you would be able to teach and to do research that enriched their own graduate training program, and so on.

Second, many faculty members' most vivid impression of you will come from the job talk, and, of course, it is impossible to deal with everything that is on each individual's mind in that context. For instance, if you didn't talk in detail about your statistical procedures, someone may be concerned about your sophistication in this area. If you did cover your statistics in great depth, someone else may wonder about your ability to teach the more theatrical, introductory lecture courses.

Given these possibilities, it makes sense to ask your host about possible reservations about your candidacy so that you can deal with them during your visit. Because this is a delicate matter, we suggest you "frame" your inquiry by asking your host to identify possible concerns that have been raised with respect to your candidacy as a result of the multiple needs of the department.

THE VISIT AND AFTER

Although departmental tribal customs for the visit vary widely, some similarities exist. Usually the visit will last at least 1 full day, perhaps a day and a half or 2 days. Try to arrive the night before your visit, get a map, and orient yourself to the campus and the town. This simple act of independence impresses faculty out of all proportion to its difficulty.

Your Host and Your Schedule. One faculty member, usually in a research area similar to your own, probably will be responsible for coordinating your visit. Your host will have your "schedule," but don't be surprised if it is not yet complete. If free time has been left on the schedule so that you can have some input, take the initiative and ask to see people or facilities of particular interest to you.

Individual Meetings. There probably will be four or five individual meetings scheduled with those faculty members who have identified themselves as being nearest your interest areas, hopefully those you researched before your visit. Double-check on them; find out what they are likely to be talking to you about and whether they have any stylistic idiosyncrasies. Do any of them believe in high-stress interviewing, for instance? You know a great deal about most of the faculty members; don't be embarrassed to ask about any new names. In the actual visits you can expect to talk about faculty members' research and some aspects of your own research. Previously you have thought about the relationship between your research and theirs; now be prepared to talk about it.

The Chairperson (and Perhaps the Dean). At this meeting, you will probably be told about the more straightforward aspects of the job, e.g., the formal fringe benefits. Here, you might also raise questions about the department's relationship with the university and get information about the "time frame" of the hiring decision—that is, how soon they will be able to make up their minds.

Talk Preparation. As soon after you arrive as possible, ask to see the room in which you are to give your talk. Don't be shocked. Frequently the room is a "temporary" one, with your slide projector set up on the some temporary "furniture." There may not be a projection screen or shades for all the windows. There may not be a podium or pointer. Don't panic, but do test the actual equipment you will use in the actual room in which you will use it. Remember that if your talk is somehow botched by the apparatus, people will "understand." However, they will not have heard you give a good talk, and you are unlikely to have the chance to do so again.

Before your talk, arrange to be off by yourself for perhaps half an hour so you can "think yourself into" what you want to say. Some departments have a tradition of a coffee hour prior to the talk; in that case, do your preparation just before the coffee hour.

Find out about certain micro-details and local talk customs. Will somebody introduce you? At the end of the talk, does someone call for questions and/or close the talk at a particular time, or are you expected to do so? Do people interrupt the talk with questions, or do they hold them until the end? If you have a relatively organized presentation, you could suggest that people hold questions until the end, unless they are unclear about some detail that would decrease their comprehension of the rest of the talk. Find out, perhaps from your host, the kind of comments to expect. Does this department have a tradition of general politeness, or do they believe in "grilling" the speaker? Be prepared to be grilled, and don't take it personally. Different traditions prevail at different institutions. Don't be surprised by them.

(As an aside to our colleagues: We have found, through trial and error, that the entire job interview goes somewhat more smoothly when candidates give their talks in the morning rather than in the usual afternoon colloquium time slot. Not only are the individual meetings facilitated by having something concrete to talk about, but the candidates themselves are less fatigued. This is especially true when candidates have flown west through several time zones the night before!)

"Social" Events. There may be a social hour after your talk and/or dinner with faculty members and/or a party after dinner. Don't be confused by the "social" nature of these events; you are still being evaluated. The faculty members are trying to discover what kind of human being you are on a wide variety of dimensions. But they are also giving you the chance to determine whether you would want to be with them. These are people with whom you are proposing to spend a lot of time. What would it feel like? Do graduate students come to these parties? What barriers seem to exist between graduate students and faculty and between junior and senior faculty? Do they seem comfortable with each other?

Drinking goes on at these events. If you drink, go ahead and join in. *But pace yourself.* Others may be able to go home early but you are the "birthday person," the guest of honor. Do know your limits, however, and leave in time to get enough sleep so that you are alert for the next day's activities.

After the Visit. You survived the visit and even enjoyed parts of it. Don't fall apart yet; there are still important details to deal with.

1. Send a list of your expenses with attached receipts to the department you visited, to the chairperson unless someone else was specifically mentioned. If at all possible, and even if it means taking out a short-term

loan, try to arrange not to be importunate about money. You will look better if you cope with this problem yourself, rather than asking for special treatment. Everybody knows that graduate students are not rich. They will process the request for payment as quickly as they can.

2. If you promised material to any faculty members during your visit, send it promptly.

3. Settle down to wait. Either the chairperson or your host might have told you when the university would probably reach a decision. In our experience, they are almost always too optimistic. If they say 2 weeks, don't be surprised to wait a month.

NOT GETTING THE JOB OFFER: HEARING NOTHING AND HEARING NO

After your wait, one of three outcomes may occur. You may get the job, fail to get it, or not hear anything about it.

Hearing No. You may get a polite letter saying that the institution you visited is not going to offer you the job. Try not to be too depressed. In our experience, it is not usually because we have a low assessment of some job candidates that we do not offer them a job. More likely we have discovered some mismatch between their talents and interests and the job, which became apparent only at the interview. Take our word for it; we are generally impressed by the job candidates we invite, even those to whom we do not offer the job.

Hearing Nothing. As you must know by now, academic decision making always takes a long time. But you should face another possibility. Because you were invited for an interview, it is clear that you are one of the best candidates for the job. However, you are certainly not the *only* good candidate. So the university may already have offered the job to another candidate. But that doesn't mean you are out of the running. If that person declines the job, it may be offered to you next but the unversity did not want to explain that you are their second choice and resolved their dilemma by not communicating with you at all. Eventually, you will probably hear from them.

GETTING THE JOB OFFER: TAKING THE JOB

Although you may find this difficult to believe, for most students, after a certain number of cycles through the search and interview process, a job offer does materialize. Then what?

It's a Job You Really Want

Let's assume you are generally enthusiastic about the institution and want to accept the job offer. Telephone them and say so. But before you finally commit yourself, resolve any questions that are important to you. Perhaps you and your spouse should make a second visit to the institution, so that you both can see where you may be spending the next few years. Determine whether the institution can cover this expense or not.

What about your contract? It will probably consist of a letter from the dean or chairperson offering you a job as an assistant professor at a certain salary. Respond with a letter accepting the job, and include a paragraph or two about issues important to you. You do this not so that you can "sue the bastards" if they fail to live up to the contract, but simply to remind them of your expectations so that they can facilitate your development. (See Bernstein, 1978, for a more complete discussion of items for contractual consideration.)

You may be able to negotiate some points with the institution, but as a person being offered your first position, you are in a poor bargaining position. Do state your needs clearly and strongly, but unless you really mean it, do not make your acceptance of the job conditional on these points. Because the department presumably wants you to be happy and productive, it may be flexible about those elements of the job that are under its control, although some aspects of the job offer, such as starting salary, tend to be set at a university-wide level.

Juggling: Being Offered the Job You Might Want

Assume a slightly more complicated set of circumstances. You have received a job offer, but not one from your "first choice" institution. You will probably be asked to reply within 2 weeks, so you had better move fast.

If you have already visited a preferred institution, you or your advisor can ask fairly directly if they want to make you a job offer. But be prepared for ambiguous responses, like "Yes, if the university approves this year's budget request," or "Yes, if Candidate X turns the job down." Neither of these answers is helpful, given the time pressure, but you can ask the institution making the offer to give you a few extra days to resolve your conflict. They may be able to do so.

If you sent your vita to an institution in which you are terribly interested, and have not been invited for a visit, your job chances are slim. But we know about closure; you may need to play this through until you find out it is not a realistic possibility. You or your advisor can call the institution and find out as much as possible about where you stand in their decision-making process. Again, the likeliest outcome is vagueness.

Given all this vagueness, it is our actuarial experience that people frequently take the first job they are offered. After pursuing all these possibilities, the bird in the hand proves considerably better than beating about bushes that may contain no birds at all.

Finishing

Congratulations! You have a job: Now retrieve your head and return to graduate school. Notice that pile of materials gathering dust in a corner? That is your thesis. *Finish it.* This may be the single most important piece of advice in this chapter. Our experience has clearly shown that the anguish associated with thesis completion goes up astronomically in attempting to do it in absentia. During your first teaching year, you will have no time to work on your thesis. Also, the role of faculty member is not well-matched with the essentially graduate student obligation of finishing a thesis. For these reasons, many students who leave with all but their degree never do get the degree. And not completing the thesis can cost you considerably. At some universities, your job will pay less and have a lesser title and you may lose it if you go too long with your thesis uncompleted. At all institutions people notice. Failure to complete the degree is a real handicap.

We have described the hiring process as we see it, but other people have other images (cf. Iacono, 1981) and you need to know about them. We hope you can use this chapter as a starting point for initiating more extensive discussions of the hiring process with your faculty advisors.

ACKNOWLEDGMENTS

We wish to thank numerous individuals who read and commented on previous drafts of the manuscript, including Jo-Anne McDowell, Thane Pittman and Shelagh Towson. Special thanks go to Phil Zimbardo whose graduate seminar on professional issues has enhanced the current version of this chapter. Earlier versions of this chapter appeared in the *Catalog of Selected Documents in Psychology,* 1979, *9,* 45-46, and in *Canadian Psychology,* 1981, *22,* 228-237.

REFERENCES

Bernstein, B. E. (1978). Points to ponder when seeking a new professional position. *Professional Psychology,* 9, 341–349.

Bryson, R. B., Bryson, J. B., Licht, M. H., & Licht, B. G. (1976). The professional pair: Husband and wife psychologists. *American Psychologist, 31,* 10–17.

Crossman, E. K., & Nazzaro, J. R. (1976). The vita. In P. J. Woods (Ed.), *Career opportunities for psychologists.* Washington, DC: American Psychological Association.

Greaves, G. B. (1979). *Securing a position in psychology: A practical guide*. Decatur, GA: Clairmont House.

Grinder, R. D. (1976). Unsolicited letters (do-it-yourself prescriptions for coping with the job shortage when you are a member of Ph.D. surplus). In P. J. Woods (Ed.), *Career opportunities for psychologists*. Washington, DC: American Psychological Association.

Iacono, W. G. (1981). The academic job interview: The experiences of a new Ph.D. in the job market. *Canadian Psychology, 22,* 217–227.

Madell, T. O., & Madell, C. M. (1979). A professional pair at the job market: A reply. *American Psychologist, 34,* 275–276.

Matthews, J. R., & Matthews, L. H. (1978). A professional pair at the job market. *American Psychologist, 33,* 780–782.

Perlman, E., & Perlman, D. (1981). The EROS principle: Giving convention papers. *Physical Therapy, 61,* 40–44.

Quereshi, M. Y. (1980). *Correlates of the employability of college/university teachers of psychology*. Paper presented at the 88th Annual Convention of the American Psychological Association, Montreal, Quebec, Canada.

Quereshi, M. Y. (1983). *Correlates of the employability of psychologists in academia: A cross-validation*. Paper presented at the 91st Annual Convention of the American Psychological Association, Anaheim, CA.

Woods, P. J. (Ed.). (1976). *Career opportunities for psychologists*. Washington, DC: American Psychological Association.

2

THE PRESENT-MINDED PROFESSOR: CONTROLLING ONE'S CAREER

Shelley E. Taylor
University of California, Los Angeles

Joanne Martin
Stanford University

As a graduate student, you may have looked forward longingly to the years when you would have the freedom to choose your own direction, set your own agenda, and embark on your day-to-day activities with no tests, papers, or other evaluations hanging over your head. Those days, you thought, would come when you became a professor.

You will be shocked to learn that being a graduate student is easy compared to being a professor. Few professors, especially few assistant professors, can afford the luxury of being absent-minded. Within a month of entering your new role, you will have double, perhaps triple, the number of demands on your time that you had when you were a student. Somehow, you have to cope with all these demands, maintain your sanity, and, during the next six or seven years, do enough fine research to earn yourself tenure at a place you would enjoy working.

Given the difficulty of these tasks, it is dismaying to realize how little most new professors know about the realities of the job. Most know something more than the inevitable elderly acquaintance of the family, who will say, "How nice that you are going to be an assistant professor. Tell me, whose assistant will you be?" Most students do leave graduate school with carefully developed research skills and, often, some teaching experience. However, most have virtually no idea of the powerful stresses and conflicting demands that are inherent in being an Assistant Professor.

This chapter is an attempt to fill this void. Our aim is to help you get control of your academic and personal life so that you use the opportunities your new role creates to realize your goals. In the hope that anticipation will be helpful, we have outlined tasks and difficulties that most Assistant Professors have to face. We try to help you get a sense of what constitutes your "fair share," what tasks you should avoid, and how you can reach forward and create opportunities for yourself. Three aspects of the transition from student to professor seem to present common dilemmas: the stressful first years, hitting your stride, and preserving a life outside of work. When we know of no clean resolutions, we discuss alternatives and hope that the knowledge that others have coped with similar problems may be of some comfort. When we know of resolutions that others have found useful, we offer them.

Such a chapter is inevitably a personal account. We have drawn on our own recollections and those of our colleagues and students. Undoubtedly, our sample of personal and second-hand experiences is biased and aspects of it will not generalize to your situation. This chapter is offered as raw material, some of which you could transform into ways of being that fit your unique situation.

THE STRESSFUL FIRST YEARS

Almost any faculty member who still remembers will tell you that the first years are very stressful. Anyone who denies this is either lying or has kept his or her expectations so low that anything seems good by comparison. The reasons for this misery are both personal and job related.

On the personal level, you are probably living in a new place, where you know almost no one. If your spouse or partner has moved with you, he or she may be coping with unemployment, a less-than-satisfactory job, or, at best, a new and challenging position. If your spouse or partner has not moved with you, the problems of commuting or adjustment may be even harder to deal with. If you have no partner, you may be trying to establish a social life. In addition to coping with loneliness at a time when you need support, you have to locate the dry cleaner, the laundromat, a place to get your hair cut, a grocery store, and a reasonable mechanic for your car (not to mention a doctor, a dentist, and maybe an accountant).

On top of all this personal strain, this time period that you had anticipated with such delight is not going as you expected. Instead of planning an exciting program of research, or writing brilliant papers, you are swamped with teaching, committee work, and other tasks that have little to do with research. You are working harder, longer, and more consistently than ever before. Yet, you leave work at night with vast numbers of seemingly crucial tasks undone. Furthermore, another month has gone by and you still haven't gotten any research started. With all these problems, it is no wonder that the first years are difficult to handle.

One of the authors remembers distinctly having the sense the first week she started as an assistant professor that "the fun was over; these people mean business." Moreover, the immediate environment can be extremely intimidating. Everyone else seems established. They know each other, it seems, and have inside jokes. They have well-oiled mechanisms called labs, they have their own theories, they have written books, graduate students have stories about them, they have real furniture and pictures on their walls, and they seem absolutely certain of how everything should be done. The fledgling assistant professor may wonder whether he or she will ever be like these others. The answer is yes, with time, and a lot of work.

Teaching Courses

The amount of time that goes into designing and teaching a course is enormous. If the course is new, or the teacher relatively inexperienced, the time demands are even greater. Most new assistant professors have to design one, two, or even more new courses simultaneously. Even those presented with an existing curriculum can rarely resist the temptation to redesign it. Often much of the course material is outside their areas of expertise. Usually, most of the time before classes start has been spent finishing a thesis, rather than preparing lectures and reading lists. To the extent that pre-class preparation has been done, it often has to be redone as the new teacher copes with the limitations of what students can learn in an hour or read in a week.

First, do not panic about the amount of time you are spending on coursework. You may not get anything else done while you are planning and delivering your first courses. Typically, no one does.

There are some things you can do to prepare. Collect course reading lists, beginning while you are still in graduate school. Study the sequence of topics, the breadth of issues covered in a single class, and estimate the page length and difficulty of reading assignments given to different kinds of students. Do not hesitate to borrow ideas for topics, readings, and discussion questions. Obviously, you should not borrow anyone's syllabus in its entirety, but drawing on four or five, and adding your own ideas, is perfectly fine.

Gauge the scope of your courses carefully. A course cannot cover every important issue in psychology. On the other hand, it is inappropriate to teach variations on your dissertation topic again and again. One of the authors' first introductory lecture courses was much too all-inclusive, while her first doctoral seminar was much too narrow. Undergraduates benefit from indepth focus just as graduate students do, and graduate students need and are entitled to as much context as undergraduates.

Typically, the first version of a course reading list covers too much material. Too many pages of reading, often at too technical a level, are assigned. Much of this material will not be read, and that which is read will often not be understood. Too many weighty issues are introduced. Under these conditions, even the most conscientious students will get confused and bogged down in detail.

It is not necessary, it is not even a good idea, to cover everything you know in a single course. Undergraduates are not graduate students, and first-year graduate students are often only 1 year away from being undergraduates. Re-examine syllabi from the best courses that you took and see the focus, limitations, and editing that is implicit in what has been omitted.

Lectures also benefit from a narrowed focus. One of the authors, in a rush of eager preparation, outlined her lectures a month before classes started. The first of these lectures got through only one quarter of that day's outline. Subsequent classes fell farther behind schedule, even though efforts were made to cover material more quickly. Examples were eliminated as redundant with the abstractions they illustrated. Time for questions was nonexistent. These lectures left students bored with a steady stream of abstractions and mystified by confusing parts of the argument. Not surprisingly, every lecture prepared before classes started had to be redone.

Good lectures are simple. It is amazing how little conceptual ground can be covered in an hour. Only three or four central points can be covered thoroughly, in part because most points should be illustrated with a vivid example. Although examples are time-consuming and may seem conceptually redundant, they are essential. Good examples captivate students' imaginations, activate their memories, and help them make the transition from abstraction to what they already know. More important, examples give students time to process and integrate what has been said. In lectures, as in readings, it is better to set a realistic limit on what you want to get across and then teach those points thoroughly.

It takes a while to ease into the teaching role. Even if you taught a great deal as a graduate student, you will undoubtedly be nervous the first day. Every assistant professor who has faced a hall full of hundreds of bored undergraduates taking a required course knows fear. Even the most skilled lecturers battle anxiety about teaching. One of Harvard's most famous lecturers throws up in the men's room before the first lecture of every semester, and sometimes on other days as well. Being nervous is nothing to be ashamed of, and it will fade with time.

No matter how good a job you do in learning how to prepare your courses, you may be fighting an uphill battle if you have too many courses to teach. Sometimes heavy teaching loads are an inescapable fact of life, but do not assume this without testing it. Your course load may be more negotiable than you think. Most colleges and universities give first-year faculty lighter loads (e.g., three courses instead of four), and you should explore if this option is available for you. Also, find out—early—what is the norm for your department. If everyone else teaches four courses, there is no reason you should teach five.

Few assistant professors are asked to teach all heavy lecture courses, so if you have agreed to teach Introductory Psychology, perhaps you shouldn't have to teach Social Psychology too. If you have agreed to take on the rigorous statistics course, perhaps you can escape a second difficult undergraduate course. If your institution has a graduate program, you should negotiate for one specialized graduate seminar, ideally two. Furthermore, no one should expect you to teach thankless courses forever. After perhaps three years of service in a course you hate, it is reasonable to expect that someone else might pick it up. Discuss these options, tactfully, with your department chair. Of all the things you can do to make your teaching more enjoyable, the best investment is the time spent negotiating a teaching load which fits your interests and priorities.

Explore, too, the possibilities of guest lecturers to ease your teaching load. Why should you spend days learning a new topic when the country's expert is down the hall? Punctuating a course with an occasional guest who can give a new perspective can be very useful for you and the students. (Understand, though, that eventually you will be expected to reciprocate with guest lectures of your own.)

You can also ease your load by involving graduate TA's, if you have any, in the course. They can assume grading responsibilities and should also be expected to give an occasional lecture, especially if it is on a topic they know well. It's good experience for the graduate student.

Finally, after developing a course, you should plan to teach it for several years. All the front-end work pays off if you have good lecture notes to work from for the next two to three years. You will want to update your notes each time you teach the course, but solid preparation when you first develop it will save valuable time down the line.

Administrative Work

As a graduate student, you may have heard vague grumblings among the faculty about time-consuming administrative duties, such as committee work. There is a most unpleasant surprise waiting for the new assistant professor: Administrative work could take up every minute of your life that isn't already consumed by designing and teaching courses.

No one ever got promoted because of committee work. This is very important to understand because administrative work has a certain attraction. There is considerable responsibility and power involved with some of these tasks, such as admissions. You can quickly feel like a "real" faculty member. Administrative work is highly visible, often appreciated (in the short term), usually easy, and therefore unthreatening. If you are nervous about getting a research program started or writing up the results of a study, you can always use voluminous amounts of committee work as your justification for procrastination.

Although doing too much committee work is not a good idea, you should do your fair share. If you don't, you will be resented. The key is to find out—early—what the norms are. Ask other faculty members how many committees they are on and how much time each one takes. Some faculty serve on large numbers of committees, but some detective work will reveal that those committees meet only once a year. Some committees consume unbelievable amounts of time (e.g., admissions, faculty search), a fact which official descriptions may downplay.

Your administrative workload is negotiable. Trade-offs are possible. An individual who does a lot of committee work at the department level should not have to serve on large numbers of university committees. If you feel you are overburdened, it is possible that people who have requested your services are unaware of how much other administrative work you are doing. Sometimes problems can be alleviated or prevented by having a word with your department chairperson about your university obligations, or by discussing your departmental obligations with the university official in charge of committee assignments.

In addition to controlling the amount of administrative work you do, learn which committees or responsibilities are important and which are not. Faculty hiring is important, as you will live with the consequences for at least three years. Graduate admissions is important. On the other hand, there are committees that are entirely unimportant. One of the authors sat on a Library Committee, which was supposed to outline faculty and student requirements for a new library. Time-consuming meetings focused on such weighty issues as layout of the rooms and numbers of study carrels. After several such meetings, the author inquired politely when the library was to be built and which of the committee members was serving as liaison with the architect's office. An embarrassed silence ensued. Finally, it was admitted that no liaison existed. The architect was developing a plan for the library without input from the committee. If you cannot escape assignment to the equivalent of a Library Committee, remember that what is not worth doing, is not worth doing well. The Library Committee met fifteen years ago, and that library has never been built.

Research: You Remember Research?

At this point you may be feeling like Katherine Anne Porter, who looked back on her years as a novelist and observed, "I think I've spent about ten percent of my energies on writing. The other ninety percent went to keeping my head above water." Given the immediate imperatives of coursework and administrative tasks, it is hard to remember that research is usually a top, if not the top, priority. By now it is clear that the research goals you set in graduate school will not be achievable in your first year or two.

Given these harsh realities, allocate your limited research time very carefully. One top priority is rewriting your thesis. You have already designed it, collected the data, and written it up once. Your thesis committee should have given you a feel for whether the study is ultimately publishable. If it is, rewrite it and submit it to a journal NOW, while it is still fresh in your mind. It will give you a sense of accomplishment and a solid empirical contribution to launch your career.

Second, consider submitting a paper for preparation at the meeting of the American Psychological Association (APA). Active involvement in these meetings is an excellent way to meet colleagues in your field from other parts of the country and there is no time like the present to start the habit. Perhaps you can slice off a piece of your thesis or present some preliminary data from another piece of work. You may feel that you have plenty of time to do this. After all, the meetings are in August. Submissions, however, are due in January. The rule for writing APA proposals is KISS (Keep It Simple, Stupid). As in outlining lectures, try to make only a few key points. Do not attempt to present complicated theoretical ideas or four-way interactions. Given the page limitations of the proposals, and the time and space limitations of symposium and poster sessions, you will not be able to communicate complexities effectively. If you attempt to do so in a proposal, the reviewers will probably turn it down. You will not need this kind of kick in the head at this stage in your career, particularly if you interpret a negative review as reflecting badly on the quality of your ideas, rather than their complexity. Avoid the problem by writing a cogent, pared-down proposal.

You should also try to get some new research going this first year, if only to convince yourself that you can do it without the help of your advisor. Starting research requires the resolution of two issues: you have to decide what to study and how to pay for it. Here are some hints on each.

You don't have to continue working on your thesis topic. It is true that you can be fairly sure your department approves of work in your thesis area, because, after all, they did hire you. It is probably also true that you feel confident of your expertise in this topic area. However, you may be bored by now with your dissertation topic. If your heart isn't in it, don't do it. One of the most important benefits of being a professor is that you have the freedom to choose what problems you work on. Exercise this right. You have earned it.

In deciding what research to do, you may wish to start by developing tests of, or tests of variants of, other people's ideas. This is relatively easy to do, it is often publishable, and it gives you exposure. However, eventually you should test your own ideas. If you want to do so immediately, and if you can express those ideas in testable form, that is all the more to your credit. Be careful not to be too grandiose. Fledgling researchers are tempted by highly abstract, multivariate theories which supposedly encompass much of the previous research in the field. Such theories seldom live up to their promise. If they do appear to, it is usually for the wrong reasons. For example, often such theories are not falsifiable. Furthermore, the stars of the field will not be overjoyed to learn that everything they have thought of during the last twenty years can be subsumed by your theory. Avoid the temptation, then, to be all-encompassing. Develop mid-range theoretical ideas that can be tested with convincing, sound, and interesting studies.

You are going to need research funds. If you have been fortunate, your institution has given you start-up funds. If not, they may be willing to do so. Many colleges and universities have faculty grants or access to specially funded programs which make small amounts of money available to faculty who fill out a brief application. This is an easy way to get started. If your institution does not offer sufficient funds to mount a longer-term research program (and most don't), you should, as soon as you can, write a grant proposal. This is a special skill, covered in Baron's chapter in this volume. Take these guidelines seriously. In addition, be sure you have someone at your institution who has received funds recently read your proposal draft. These safeguards may save you considerable time and heartache.

To write an article based on your thesis, submit a paper to APA, plan one study (and hopefully run it), and prepare a funding proposal. This may seem to be a very modest set of research goals. If you can manage more, fine. But, before you tackle other projects, be sure you've finished these four tasks. Few get that far in the first year. Besides, in doing these things, you should also save some time for establishing good relationships with the faculty and students in your department.

Reading: Staying on Top of the Field

A not-so-famous psychologist once said, "You can be a reader or a writer, but not both." He changed from being a reader to being a writer and shortly thereafter became more famous. His point is well taken. The volume of research that is generated in the field is enough to keep one, maybe two or three, individuals reading full-time.

Reading the *Journal of Personality and Social Psychology, JPSP* (or the comparable bible in your field) cover to cover is not a good use of your time. Focus on articles germane to your classes and research interests. Do not restrict your reading to published work. By the time a paper actually appears in print, its author is at least a year or two away from it and into other studies. If you base your research only on what you see in print, you will fall behind the field. Early in your career, write to the eight or ten most influential people in your area of interest, and ask for preprints of their most recent work. If someone writes a paper in your area which you think is impressive, write the author and ask to be put on his or her mailing list, so you will receive unpublished manuscripts as soon as they are written. Scan the APA program for early versions of soon-to-be published, exciting ideas and studies. (Be selective, though. The overwhelming majority of APA presentations sound interesting, but are not worth your time.)

When you read, read for a purpose. Such purposes include planning the introduction to an article or grant, teaching, deciding how to design a study, or conducting a review of the literature. Information is best learned and retained when there is something to hang it on, and a purpose gives you that hanger. Otherwise, the information may pass right through you undigested.

Faculty Colleagues

On a professional level, colleagial relationships are both more and less than they are cracked up to be. It is a myth that colleagues gather regularly, or even irregularly, to debate weighty issues with intelligence and wit. On-going, rewarding conversations with colleagues about work-related issues are rare. On the other hand, colleagues can influence your work substantially, through such channels as casual conversations, co-teaching, colloquium presentations, sharing papers, and working with the same doctoral students.

Do try to learn from your colleagues. Many of them are brilliant, thoughtful scholars who have much to offer you. If such a person is giving a talk, go! If he or she is giving a seminar on his or her current research, strongly consider sitting in, at least occasionally. You may be rewarded with insight, profundity, and even friendship.

It is tempting to pitch your work towards your departmental colleagues, not pursuing ideas that are greeted with skepticism and following up on suggestions which are tangential to your interests. After all, your colleagues will be determining whether you will retain your present position. Ultimately, however, your stature in the field depends on a far wider audience. Feedback from local colleagues is important, but even the most eminent and wise individuals represent only a tiny part of the entire field.

Sometimes a colleague will give you a paper to critique. Be flattered, but circumspect. Doing a lengthy, constructive critique for a colleague may help him or her and make you look smart. But, perhaps the colleague didn't want criticism—perhaps he or she wanted your flattery and/or gratitude. Try to discern the colleague's goal and temper your feedback with this knowledge.

Junior faculty often have to decide whether to accept a senior colleague's offer of collaboration. There are obvious benefits to such collaboration. It is flattering to be asked and your work might well be importantly enriched. However, the risks of such collaboration are substantial. The results of your joint endeavors are likely to be credited to your senior colleague, not to you, even if the ideas are clearly yours. Even if the behavior of your senior colleague is exemplary, others in the field may fail to give you credit, recognition, and, ultimately, tenure for the work. Once you have established your reputation as a scientist in your own right, collaboration with colleagues, even eminent senior colleagues, is perfectly all right—even highly desirable. However, too much collaboration with senior people, too early in your career, places you at great risk.

On the other hand, you should not err too far in the other direction. Many of your colleagues genuinely want to help you and you should let them. They have been professors longer than you and know how your institution works. They will undoubtedly be able to tell you useful things. Offers to read paper drafts and grant proposals can be especially helpful, saving time and embarrassment. This is not to say that you should camp on your colleagues' doorsteps, whimpering for assistance every other day. But, if someone is willing to give an occasional spot of advice about a tough dilemma, accept it with gratitude.

Assistant professors often have the impression that their progress is being monitored on an almost daily basis by their colleagues. This is certainly not true. Neither are they shunning you. They may well be leaving you alone to give you a chance to get settled. They are busy and only dimly aware of the day-to-day activities of people in the department. No matter how fascinating you are, rest assured that you are not a major focus of their attention. So, do not be paranoid. Remember, one of the reasons your colleagues hired you was that they felt you would be someone they would enjoy and get along well with.

Do not prove them wrong. Be sure you take the time to have fun with your colleagues. Have lunch, go for drinks, accept and return invitations to dinner, play softball in the spring and squash in the winter, and/or attend informal departmental gatherings. An unnerving amount of university business is conducted in these settings, and so it is important that you be there. But more important, you will have a good time, it will make you feel more relaxed, you will make some good friends, and you will understand that your colleagues are people too.

Early on, you should realize that there is a phenomenon called department and university politics. The collective history of everything that happened before you got there stays around in various formal and informal ways. Certain factions in the department may be warring with each other. Certain professors may dislike each other intensely. Personality conflicts may be played out over seemingly objective issues like space allocation or faculty slots.

The main thing to be said about department politics is: Don't be stupid. Don't take strong stands on issues you don't understand immediately after arriving at the university. Keep your ear to the ground, listen carefully, ask questions, and figure out as much of the politics as you can. You do not want to offend people inadvertently. You may choose to offend them at some later point, when you understand the dimensions of the issue, but to do so in error is foolish.

Usually, after six or eight months at an institution (longer for those of us who tend to be oblivious to such issues), you will have picked up enough of what is going on through faculty meetings, informal conversations with colleagues, scuttlebutt from fellow junior faculty, and the like to understand both the explicit and implicit agendae that are being played out in your department. At that point, you are in a position to take informed stances or to remain neutral, as you choose.

Working with Students

One of the most important aspects of one's role as an assistant professor is working individually with students. This task epitomizes many of the reasons people become professors. Your role as an educator is paramount, and you are working under ideal conditions: imparting the basic skills of the discipline by working one-on-one with a student whom you have had a voice in selecting. You are also epitomizing your role as a researcher, as this is generally the direct or indirect focus of your work with the student. Finally, by working on research with a student you are acknowledging the collaborative nature of the scientific endeavor. Given the centrality of these issues, the act of taking on a student engenders important obligations—to yourself and to the student.

It is crucial, to select students very carefully. When you first begin your new job, you may sit for hours in your office praying that a student will knock on your door and say, "I want to work with you." Accordingly, when someone finally does, you are inclined to say yes immediately. You may be lucky with this approach, but you may also get a loser. You might, for example, have taken on the person that no one else wants to work with.

Before you establish a firm commitment, you should make some inquiries. If you are dealing with graduate students, intelligence should not be your primary criterion for selection. Most students who get into graduate school are at least fairly bright. Although some level of intelligence is essential for success in graduate school, lack of intelligence is seldom the primary obstacle to a student's becoming a productive researcher. Instead, the typical obstacles include procrastination, perfectionism, too many interests, and disorganization. When you make inquiries about a student, try to find out what that student's fatal flaw might be and then take steps, in advance, to keep it from getting in the way.

You may be collaborating with undergraduates, either because your institution does not have a graduate program or by preference, because the undergraduates are unusually good. Typically, good undergraduate research assistants are bright, conscientious, and enthusiastic, and have a comprehensive ignorance of the process of doing research. Undergraduates can be great workers, but left to their own devices, they will often mess up a perfectly good research idea because they are unaware of the right way to solve a problem. Even with the brightest of undergraduates, you must be prepared to invest your time in training and supervision. This is inevitably a time-consuming process. Generally, undergraduate research assistants work out best doing well-defined tasks on projects that are already underway. Often a graduate student can supervise the undergraduate's work. This can free your time, be a valuable educational experience for the undergraduate, and provide the graduate student with important supervisory experience, as well as help on a project or pilot data collected in an area of mutual interest.

Once you have selected students, the next problem is supervising them. At least three mistakes are common. The first is over-supervision, particularly of advanced graduate students. People are in graduate school because they are bright enough and experienced enough to bear some responsibility for their own work. If you treat graduate students like undergraduates, and supervise every detail of their work, you can expect them to resent you and want to work with other professors who will keep them on a looser rein.

A second common mistake is related to the first. A faculty member should not insist that a student work on the faculty member's project in precisely the way the faculty member has anticipated. Even the apprenticeship model of graduate education does not justify this approach, which makes shabby use of a fine student mind. Although the impetus and direction of a research project may lie with the faculty member, students should have an opportunity to make creative contributions. Otherwise, the potential benefits of collaboration are lost to both participants.

A third common mistake in the process of supervision is to delegate too much to the student. It makes no sense to hand a project over to a student, expecting to receive keypunched data some weeks later. The project will almost certainly not be executed in the manner which you expect. Unanticipated obstacles always arise, either in the design or execution. The results may be expensive and unpublishable, leaving you gravely disappointed. It is possible to delegate a large percentage of the work on a project to a student, but frequent meetings (weekly, even biweekly) are essential. At these meetings you can assess whether all parts of the project are progressing smoothly, make revisions as necessary, and, in the process, give the student the prompt and specific feedback which should be an integral part of this kind of educational relationship. These issues are covered in more detail in Zanna and Darley's chapter in this volume.

Making Ends Meet

An unhappy fact about our profession is that it pays very little, particularly in the early years. It barely supports a swinging singles life style, and pushes the edge of the poverty line for a family. In fact, a colleague of one of the authors was informed, to his shock, that his children were eligible for their school's free hot lunch program because their family's income was so low. Because moneymaking opportunities arise from time to time, it is tempting to take these on.

When you are deciding whether or not to take on a moneymaking venture, think about three things: How much money will it actually make you for the time invested? How much time will it take? Are there any professional advantages? Your discretionary thinking time in your job is low, perhaps no more than a fifth or a quarter of your total working time. Therefore, to clutter it up with moneymaking tasks that bring you no professional rewards can truly do you a disservice.

Beware the lump sum. Most people grossly underestimate the amount of time it takes them to do any project. Therefore, a lump sum of $200, say, for reviewing a textbook may look great. A week later, when you are still organizing your comments for a typist, you may regret that you took on this particular task. Consulting on an hourly basis with a business organization is frequently lucrative. However, it may also be time-consuming and may take you away from your professional agenda. Your publication record may fall off, and ultimately, you may have gained short-term financial aid at the expense of long-term prospects for tenure.

A chance to write textbooks (or a section of a textbook) often comes one's way. The amount of time that goes into such an endeavor (when one includes initial writing, rewriting, going over copyedited manuscripts and galleys, and reference location) can be enormous. The professional payoffs are few, and the royalty figure may be somewhat lower than was initially estimated.

Another way that faculty members sometimes supplement their income is by teaching courses in summer school. Again, you may need to do this for financial reasons, but there are also risks. Summer is one of the few times when the work pace slows down, when you have a chance to do some writing and thinking. You begin to remember why you entered this profession. If you fill up the summer with the same kinds of obligations you have during the year, you may burn yourself out. To the extent that you can avoid these activities and still keep your head above the water, try to protect your free time so you can do some high quality thinking. But if you must take on moneymaking tasks, do try to make them ones that are truly lucrative, that can help rather than hinder your career, and that do not end up taking all of your discretionary time.

If You Are a Minority Group Member or a Woman

If you are not a white male, you will probably have an extra dose of all the difficulties described above. For example, you may be expected to teach a course on the Psychology of X's (where X equals your group, i.e., Hispanics, blacks, women). This may happen even if this topic is unrelated to your areas of academic specialization. Undoubtedly, you will be asked to carry an unusually heavy load of administrative work. Every committee seems to feel it needs to have an X, and the fewer the X's around, the more likely it is that you will be contacted. In addition to these demands on your time, you will be bombarded with a myriad of requests from publishers, colleagues, students, and journalists to speak or write about potentially explosive or personally impolitic topics, such as "Prejudice in Our School" or "Difficulties of Being a Pregnant Professor."

Simply because you are a member of an under-represented group does not mean that you have to teach courses outside your area of expertise, carry an extraordinarily heavy administrative workload, or speak publicly about prejudice or your private life. You can say no. There is a stereotype that minorities and women are unable to do good, substantive empirical and theoretical work. If you spend too much of your time away from your research, you will feed this stereotype. No one will remember the other things you have been doing.

It is difficult to decide when to say no. When a committee chairperson calls you to say, in despairing tones, that the committee needs an X to represent the X point of view, ask your self: Is this true? Is a woman really needed to help with the allocation of secretarial services? Is a black really necessary on curriculum revision committee? Maybe so, but then again, maybe not. And even if an X is necessary, need you be that X? Pick your acceptances very carefully. If you feel that your status as an X will really make a critical contribution, say yes, but be sure you get off something else in exchange.

Even using these guidelines for choosing acceptances, you will still have more invitations than you can accept without seriously cutting into your research time. One of the authors has developed a four-yeses-per-month rule. That rule means as many as 40 no's per month.

There will be times when you will not want to say no. For example, student X's, who have been waiting years for an X on the faculty, now have you to turn to. They may want to work with you because you must be interested in the Psychology of X's, because they are more comfortable with an X, because they want an X as a role model, or because they have personal or academic difficulties that stem, in part, from being an X. Many of these reasons are completely legitimate.

However legitimate these reasons are, you cannot let yourself be swamped by X students. You do not want a reputation as a faculty member who works only with X's, not Y's or Z's. On the other hand, you will want to say yes to some X's. Making these choices is painful. Some of the students who want to study the Psychology of X will have to be sent to a Y advisor, even though you suspect that Y will not have the slightest idea what the study is all about. Students who want to work with you because you are an X, rather than because you have similar intellectual interests, should probably be sent to someone else. Some of the students with personal problems will have to be sent to a mental health service, however poor that service may be. You cannot be all things to all X's and you do not want to be a representative X in all your activities. Nevertheless, some of these negative decisions, particularly about students, will be difficult to make.

In addition to these extra demands on your time, if you are one of a very few members of your demographic group, you may have other, more serious problems to cope with. You may encounter blatant prejudice, as when one of the authors was seated with the faculty wives, rather than the professors, at a luncheon for a visiting dignitary.

Sometimes the prejudice surfaces in more subtle and potentially dangerous forms. For example, you may find that people's expectations about your performance are either too high (the few who expect you to be a shining example, outperforming all others) or too low (the many who believe that X's seldom exceed mediocrity). The people whose expectations are sky-high will be disappointed when they find out that you are human. Low expectations may be resistant to change, even when evidence of superior performance is clear. Worse yet, if low expectations are widespread and resistant to change, you may find they have a detrimental effect on your performance. Your faith in your own abilities can be seriously undermined.

Under these conditions, it is very hard for you to distinguish accurate from positively or negatively biased feedback. You wouldn't want to blame yourself for negative feedback that was merely the result of prejudice. You wouldn't want to blame prejudice when the real fault was in the quality of your own work. It is essential to find people who will give you honest, critical, unbiased feedback.

Sometimes you may feel socially isolated. You may get asked to lunch less frequently than your non-X colleagues, and you may be less likely to be tapped for a squash game. As noted above, these informal contacts with colleagues can be a valuable source of information, and so women and minorities may be inadvertently left out of these opportunities for exchanging information.

Parties may also be awkward. For example, one of the authors and her husband walked into a cocktail party where the faculty spouses, all females, were standing in one corner, talking about the best place to buy children's rubber boots, while the male professors were in the other corner, avidly discussing university politics. Should a male faculty spouse join the faculty wives? Should a female faculty member join the all-male faculty group? Feeling ill at ease in social situations, such as this party, can impede development of comfortable relations with your colleagues. The help of a few sensitive individuals can really make a difference. At the party described above, a tactful male colleague called out a greeting and walked forward to create a mixed group that quickly expanded, dramatically changing the conversational dynamics for the rest of the party.

You may find that you have to take the initiative to make up for a dearth of informal contacts. If no one asks you to play squash, then sharpen your skills, call a colleague, and make a squash date. Or, take the initiative and invite a colleague who has interesting ideas about a particular issue out to lunch. If you are a woman, these gestures will occasionally be misinterpreted, but a friendly businesslike attitude, free of sexual innuendo, should create the appropriate climate relatively quickly.

People may find it hard to believe that an X can be an Assistant Professor. One dismal morning, one of the authors was mistaken for an undergraduate, a secretary, the person responsible for watering plants, and a cashier. For females, answering your own telephone may cause considerable confusion until the caller understands that you are the professor, not the professor's secretary. Even when people have learned that you are indeed a professor, they may address you by your first name, while referring to other faculty as "Dr." or "Professor." These cases of mistaken identity are each trival, but the repeated incidence of such episodes clearly communicates a sense that the world considers it unlikely, if not illegitimate, for you to be an Assistant Professor.

These kinds of problems recur day after day, year after year. Generally, the perpetrators mean well and are not being intentionally prejudiced. In fact, if you were to confide in them about any one of these incidents, they would probably produce a credible alternate explanation which has nothing to do with prejudice. Furthermore, they may ask if, perhaps, you aren't being a bit over-sensitive?

It is all too easy to get a reputation as an oversensitive complainer about these issues. You are the only one who knows how often such incidents occur; these kinds of things don't often happen to non-X's. Furthermore, an alternative, non-prejudiced explanation for some of these incidents may be correct. However, remember parsimony. If a dozen incidents can be explained by a dozen alternative explanations or by a single hypothesis about prejudice, have faith in your judgment.

This does not mean that you should share your convictions about the prevalence of prejudice with large numbers of others. You might decide to talk about these incidents only at "teachable moments," keeping your discomfort to yourself when speaking up would do no good. Given the frequency of prejudicial incidents in some institutions, this strategy might mean that you would have to swallow too much anger, confusion, and frustration for your own good. Another strategy is to find a few, carefully selected confidants. You could also let off steam by speaking up to perpetrators, not only at "teachable moments," but also when you need to, for your own mental health. After all, the best thing you can do for yourself, and for the group of which you are a member, is to give yourself the time and mental strength you need to do your job, as you define it, as well as you can.[1]

The best thing about the stressful first years is that eventually, and often gradually, they end. You lose your obsession with coursework and committees. Panic, at the amount of work you have to do, begins to subside. You begin to hit your stride. You begin to feel competent and to remember all those reasons why you wanted to become a professor in the first place.

HITTING YOUR STRIDE

Hitting your stride in academic worklife is primarily a matter of settling on a research strategy and learning to manage your limited time efficiently. We will begin with research strategy, since this provides the foundation for your other activities. (The comments in this section assume that research is the main criterion for tenure at your school. It is, for most major universities and many colleges as well. However, some schools honestly do not care about research productivity, and instead make tenure decisions on the basis of teaching and service. If your institution is one of these schools, and you should know by now if it is, then these comments will not fit for you.)

Research Priorities: Or, What Not To Publish

At the age of 42, to pick a random age, some researchers are still churning out interesting journal articles that are unrelated to each other. While there are rewards for this type of research in the first years of your career, those rewards eventually disappear. If you continue with this pattern of publications, you will get a reputation for being atheoretical. In order to prepare for tenure, you need to carve out a piece of the field as your own. Accordingly, 2 or 3 years into your Assistant Professorship, you should be refining your own theoretical ideas and formally testing them through a series of interrelated studies.

Having chosen a theoretical area of concentration, you should select your publication priorities carefully. First, focus on top-quality empirical publications in leading journals. At this time in your career, you will be judged primarily by the quality of the research you do, and by empirical publications in particular. The payoffs from publications in secondary journals are much lower, but they may be worthwhile, particularly if you are committed to having a certain paper see the light of day or if your co-authors are students, for whom such a publication could be particularly helpful.

In addition, try to make a strong theoretical contribution to your piece of the field. The premier publication outlet for this kind of work is an article in *Psychological Review*. Such a publication typically includes data, as well as some careful and innovative thinking about a problem, thus testifying to your strengths as both a researcher and a theoretician. To publish an article in *Psychological Bulletin* is also good. Generally, such a publication does not involve data collection, and the theoretical content is more likely a novel perspective on an established area, rather than an innovative theoretical analysis of a problem.

Chapters are a mixed blessing. You will have considerable freedom to say what you want to say, and editors will often agree in advance to let you approach a topic in an unorthodox way. Book editors, in comparison to journal editors, often have less stringent or narrowly defined standards for accepting manuscripts. Everyone knows this, so they sometimes discount chapters as publications. Avoid doing too many chapters early in your career and pick the few you do with care. A chapter can be useful if you have some good theoretical ideas and no readily available outlet for their development. If you choose to do a chapter for these reasons, select a book put out by a major publisher. The topic should be relatively broad and preferably hot. You are looking for exposure, so you do not want your chapter to sink along with a book that sells only a few hundred copies. On the other hand, you will benefit far more from a chapter which reaches a relatively small group of researchers in your field, than from exposure to larger numbers of undergraduates or practitioners. Overall, if you are going to write a chapter, make sure it's good and published in a good place. DO NOT publish slight variants of the same chapter in two (or more) places. People notice and they will be unimpressed.

Edited books, like chapters, are a mixed blessing. It is nice for you, and your proud parents, to see a book with your name on it. On the other hand, you do not get to be a primary force in shaping the ideas in the book and you may have to do a lot of intellectually undemanding and often unpleasant work (nagging, editing) to get it out. If you include chapters of your own, they may be discounted as publications by others because, after all, it is your book. If you do an edited book, make sure it's one you can be proud of.

There are some other things you should not publish early in your career. Writing textbooks may make you some money, but it is not an effective way to get ahead in the field. Writing parts of textbooks is also not an optimal use of your time. You don't get the satisfaction of organizing the field in your own way, you don't make much money, and you get little, if any, recognition for your work. Book reviews can also be an unrewarding business. Few people read book reviews. Positive reviews tend to be bland, while negative reviews make you enemies. Of course, if you are going to read the book anyway and really want to write a review, go ahead, but be warned.

Before sending your manuscript out for review, you should get feedback on it. This is particularly important early in your career. Your papers are likely to be too long, too detailed, and not clearly written. It is helpful to cultivate a couple of close colleagues, either at your own university or elsewhere, to give you critical feedback on your manuscripts. These may be friends from graduate student days, your former advisor, or simply people in your research area with whom you have developed a working relationship. Obviously, the reason people will be willing to provide this service for you is because they expect you to provide it in return. Although it will be time-consuming, it will be worth it. Often an exciting piece of research is rejected from a journal solely on the basis of how it is presented. Once you have received a rejection, there may be no way of resubmitting, even though you know that many of the flaws will be correctable. Revise and resubmit is an open door. Out-and-out rejection usually is not. Therefore, be sure you spend the time getting a manuscript in good shape before you submit it.

One observation about publications underlies all those above. There is no such thing as a quick and easy publication. Everything takes time, and time spent on one thing might be better spent on something else.

Writing

All this talk about publications assumes you have written something. Learning to write well and to enjoy the process may be one of the most difficult obstacles you face. Although writing is covered, in part, in Bem's chapter in this volume, we offer some observations here. Writer's block is a tremendous problem for many fledgling and not-so-fledgling academics. Often the problem is not that writing isn't getting done, but that no writing is perfect enough to be sent out. Endless revisions, seeking an illusory perfection, can result in a writing style that is crabbed and defensive. It is better to err on the side of sending things out prematurely, than to hold on to a draft for months or years, until is it out-of-date or stale.

Sometimes the problem is that you simply aren't spending enough time writing. When the author Colette was young, her husband locked her into her study each day. You can use figuratively similar tricks on yourself. One method of getting going is to write up a study as a convention paper first. These are usually less threatening, and the feedback received can improve subsequent writing and/or alert you to the need for a follow-up study before you submit to a journal. Or, you can get yourself to tackle a tough paper by thinking, "It's just a rough draft no one will ever see." A prominent psychologist reports that an assistant professor came up to him once to thank him profusely for teaching him how to write. "What did I do?" exclaimed the astonished psychologist. "I saw you writing on blue paper, and realized that by writing on blue paper you could think of your writing as preliminary. I had always been writing on white paper and feeling that the writing therefore had to be fully polished. When I switched to blue paper, my productivity increased enormously."

Regardless of how we trick ourselves into writing, the fact is that we simply must write. Break the paper down into sections. Start on an easy section, such as Methods. Set rewards for yourself. If you finish a particularly difficult part, perhaps you deserve a nice lunch with a friend. Alternate hard tasks with easy ones, so that a tough paper is followed by a simple revision. You may need some fallow time between papers. If you cannot start one paper immediately after finishing another, give yourself a day of reading—but select reading germane to your next paper.

It is important to figure out what conditions you need to establish the habit of writing. One of the authors needs long periods of full concentration, and so she schedules full days of writing time. This approach has the advantage of minimizing the amount of time which is lost during startups. The other author prefers to write for two or three hours every day. This method has the advantage of minimizing the amount of time you lose on those inevitable "bad days," when no words come easily. It is hard, at first, to discipline yourself to create specified times to write, but gradually writing on a schedule gives you a rhythm and teaches you how to write. It is the single most helpful thing you can do, if you are struggling with writer's block.

Whichever writing method you choose, you must allocate a minimum of about 10 hours a week for writing. If you allocate less, you simply cannot get the work done. Treat your scheduled writing time as sacred. Accept no interruptions. One of the authors has become famous for her threatening "Do Not Disturb Until 11:45" signs. Finally, before you quit writing on any given day, outline the first half-hour of the next day's writing. It will help you get started again.

Machines, like dictaphones and word processors, can help you write more efficiently. If you are fortunate enough to have a full-time or part-time secretary, invest time in learning how to dictate. Ultimately, you will save a substantial amount of time. Start with short letters, memos, and comments to students on their papers. Gradually, work up to sections of papers. For example, the methods section is often easiest to dictate. It takes about 2 or 3 weeks of regular use to learn how to dictate effectively. For the first week or so, you will actually lose time. It is important to realize this, so you will not give up prematurely.

Word processing can also be an immense time saver and it may also improve the quality of your writing. It is not necessary to know how to type. Even two-finger "hunt and peck" typists find an immediate pay-off from learning to use a word processor. Don't fear that you will waste your time doing things you currently delegate to a secretary. Even if your secretary does not have access to your word processor, even if your secretary has to retype the final version of a paper, the time you save simply on drafts will be worth it. The software programs for word processing are easy to master. Within hours, you will be saving yourself time. After a month of instantly available, clean copies of drafts, you will wonder how you ever lived without your word processor.

Access to a word processor may cost you money. A few colleges and universities make these tools available to faculty, usually by supplying access to a word processing program, a terminal, and computer time on a shared machine. When that machine goes down, you cannot write. When this happens repeatedly and unexpectedly, the frustration can be immense. The investment in your own microcomputer, also usable for data analysis, may well be worth it.

Getting Reviews

Once you learn to write and dare to submit what you have written, you have opened Pandora's box. Inevitably, you will get reviews. Steel yourself, as reviews can be a most unpleasant experience. They are sometimes hostile. You must believe the percentages that indicate that 85% or 95% of the papers at certain journals get rejected. Everyone gets rejections, and you will be no exception.

One of your first reactions may be fury. How could the reviewers and editor have missed seeing the brilliance of your work? Write a furious letter to them, if you must, but please don't mail it. You will be submitting papers to this journal or to these people again. Instead, decide right away what you want to do next.

Some researchers take a rejected paper and put it immediately in the mail to another journal. We think, instead, that it is smarter to take advantage of the criticisms you have received. In some cases, suggestions for revisions or replications will be well-taken and will foreshadow comments you will get from reviewers elsewhere. There is always the danger you will get the same reviewers, who will not be pleased to see their pearls of wisdom ignored.

If your paper has been rejected with encouragement to resubmit, by all means, do so soon. You should plan to address every major criticism raised by the editor and the reviewers. Either modify the coverage in the paper or explain in a cover letter why you chose not to. Writing such cover letters is an art form. Your objective should be to save the editor work. You may be delighted that your revised paper varies from the old one in numerous ways. The editor, however, will react with dismay because it is hard to see how you have responded to all the criticisms. In your cover letter, highlight briefly where each of the major problems was addressed. The editor will be extremely grateful and your manuscript may be processed more quickly.

Sometimes, a manuscript will be rejected by two or three journals. Do not keep resubmitting it indefinitely. If one journal has found a fatal flaw in your study, chances are that a reviewer at another journal will do the same. In any case, the payoff for publishing your article in an obscure place is probably not worth the time it would take for you to do another revision. Eventually, bite the bullet. Put the article in the back of your file drawer and stop throwing good time after bad. Go on to something else.

Providing Reviews

Once you begin to publish, you will not only be getting reviews of your work, but also be asked to provide them for others. At first, it is difficult to know how to review a manuscript. Fledgling reviewers tend to pick at grammar and spelling, ignoring the more important points. To see what kind of information goes into a review, read a lot of reviews. Look at your own carefully. Ask your graduate student advisor if he or she would be willing to let you see other reviews, so you can get a sense of how good ones are written.

Once the fledgling reviewer overcomes the problem of what to put in a review, he or she tends to turn nasty. Resist this temptation. Once you have found a flaw in a manuscript, refrain from adopting a tone that clearly conveys your sense that this author is a moron who should no longer be permitted to practice science. Realize, first, that the author has spent a great deal more time thinking about this problem than you have, and may well have thought of your criticism, but not have written about it well. If there is indeed a flaw in the manuscript, point it out, but do so in a way that does not impugn the writer's character. Think of a review as an opportunity for constructive feedback. How could the author improve the work or design a Study Two to remedy the flaws in the first study? In short, view reviewing as an opportunity for anonymous scientific interchange, not a license to vent hostility.

As you advance in your career, you will find yourself increasingly asked to provide reviews. Indeed, you could spend much of your professional time providing them. A good review takes at least several hours, even after one has a lot of experience, and this is a startlingly large portion of the discretionary time that one has available to oneself in a week. A useful rule of thumb is not to accept more than two reviews at any given time. If you are providing more than 20 reviews a year, then you are probably reviewing too much.

Self-Promotion

If you have planned your research strategy and gotten out a couple of papers, and you are still waiting to be discovered, don't hold your breath. No one is going to discover you: you have to promote yourself. Your advisors hopefully have brought you to the attention of their colleagues, by writing rave letters about you and by introducing you at conferences. Now, they have other students they are introducing and you are left on your own. It is not inappropriate, rude, pushy, or aggressive to promote yourself. It is standard operating procedure. So, how do you market your work?

First, if you have a paper you are particularly proud of, send it to people in the field. Don't just send it to your mother and your graduate school buddies. Don't be afraid to send it to people whose work is important and relevant to your own. Send it to people whose work you cited. These are the colleagues who are most likely to be interested in, to profit from, and ultimately to cite your work. They are also the individuals who, one way or another, will evaluate it.

Do what you can to increase the chances that people will read what you send them. Do not send out everything you write. Most people have very little time to read. They will be far less interested in a fat envelope, containing four papers, than in a single, solid piece published or to-be-published in a leading journal. Accompany the paper with a personal note, explaining how the paper might be of interest to the recipient. Understand, however, that three quarters of the recipients will chuck your beloved paper in the circular file. A few will read it, they may cite it, and eventually your work will start to be known. Send the paper to people in the research area, to people writing books that will cover work like yours, and to authors of Annual Review of Psychology chapters or their equivalents. These strategies increase the chances that your work will be cited.

When should you send out a paper? The pre-prints stage is a good time. Because a paper is "in press," it has been peer-reviewed and revised. Consequently, its rough edges are gone. Moreover, it is "hot"—not yet out, but hopefully soon to be influential. Pre-publication drafts are okay to send, if they're polished and you want the feedback. And, reprints are important to send, so that people will have the final, slim, version for their files.

Talk about your work. Give brown bag lunches, colloquia, and conference presentations. Do not sit around waiting for someone to invite you to be on an APA symposium. Think up a symposium topic that would be well-timed and well-received, and organize a symposium yourself. It would undoubtedly be nice to invite as panelists your graduate student friends who are now assistant professors, scattered all over the country. Avoid this temptation, as such a symposium is unlikely to attract a strong audience. Try to find panelists who are doing well-regarded work in the area. Do not be afraid to call up senior scientists in the field, asking them to present papers or be discussants. What harm can it do to ask? Even famous people sometimes have to be on the APA program to get their expenses paid. Be prepared for the fact that they may want to be chairs or discussants, rather than presenters. In any case, simply by calling them, you have increased the chances that they will remember you and your work.

Give others opportunities to get to know you and to promote themselves by inviting them to give colloquia or brown bag lunches in your department. In particular, invite prominent people who are in your field. They will be flattered by your interest, and your own colleagues may think better of your work by seeing the exemplary work of the best people in your field. Who knows, you may even be mentioned during the talk! It can't hurt.

It may seem discouraging that in academia, as in business, a certain amount of self-promotion is done. Professors don't just do their research and publish it, they market their ideas. If you do not participate in these activities, it will not be fatal, but it will impede somewhat the development of your career. Besides, getting to know the people in your field, and having discussions focused on your ideas, can be a great pleasure.

Time Management

The longer you stay in a field, the more people will know who you are, and the more work will pile up on your desk. Letting your workload get out of control can literally kill you, it can make your worklife pretty miserable, and it can make your personal life non-existent. You can get control of your workload if, and only if, you are willing to be ruthless with yourself about the way you use your time.

"Ruthless" is a strong word. Before proceeding, we should admit that the authors are outliers when it comes to planning and time management. We were both making detailed plans by the age of eight. We have both been known to carry as many as five "to do" lists, classified by type of task and date of deadline.

Notwithstanding our perhaps over-zealous stance on these issues, the time demands on professors' time are impossible. If you don't make your priorities clear to yourself and others, if you aren't willing to sacrifice spontaneity for planning, if you don't learn to plan realistically, you are hurting yourself. When you have worked out priorities, plans, and a time schedule, you don't let time slip through your fingers. You know just what to do, and what can be done, in an unanticipated half hour. You are less likely to disappoint yourself, because you have a realistic idea of what you can accomplish in a given time period. Finally, you are also less likely to disappoint others, by making commitments you cannot keep.

We offer some suggestions about getting organized and managing time in the academic setting. You should also know that there are several good time management/organization books that are helpful in this regard. Two we recommend are Alan Lakein's *How to Get Control of Your Time and Your Life* and Alec MacKenzie's *The Time Trap*. They may seem a little strange in their single-minded, urgent preoccupation with time, but they are full of many helpful suggestions.

Establishing Priorities

The first step in effective planning is establishing your priorities. Your research plans should be your chief guide, so focus on the area of research you have chosen to carve out as your own. Give your highest priority to empirical projects, supplemented by one or two theoretical pieces. Next come projects that are near completion and those which you feel irrevocably, morally committed to complete. Third come projects that you might like to undertake sometime in the future, but to which, if you had been wise, you have not yet made a formal commitment.

It is useful to have some kind of organizational device that keeps your priorities firmly in mind. For one colleague, this is simply a stack of 21 nine-inch-wide and one-inch-high pigeonholes with names of projects, students, and courses written on them. One of the authors keeps a manila file of goals, organized into high, medium, and low priorities. You should develop a system that works for you.

Using the Pipeline

Organize your research life so that it has a continuous, temporal flow. At all times, you should have projects at all parts of the pipeline. Some projects will be in the formulative problem stage, whereas others will be in the design, data collection, data analysis, writing, or review phases. You may only have one project at each of these stages of development, but keeping the pipeline filled at each stage keeps all your skills active, enables you to be consistently productive, gives you a variety of research tasks to do, and gives a flow to your work. The pipeline approach is easy to use if you have developed an interrelated set of ideas on one general topic. As the findings from the first study become clear, you will know how to modify the theory and design for the second study. Results from completed studies can also enable you to refine your research priorities and eliminate projects that are no longer desirable or significant parts of your work.

From Priorities to Task Statements and Time Estimates

Most poor planners make three kinds of mistakes. First, they fail to be specific enough, saying "write JPSP article," rather than "write Methods section on Tuesday morning." Second, they are over-optimistic about time estimates, again and again. As a result, they are repeatedly disappointed in themselves and in the planning process. And, third, poor planners often fail to delegate wherever possible. This problem is particularly acute for academics. As a group, we tend to be loners and, automatically, to do everything ourselves, rather than investing the time it takes to train others, such as secretaries, graduate students, and work-study students.

It is possible to avoid these mistakes. For each of your top priority projects, split the remaining work into tasks, such as designing a questionnaire, pre-testing subjects, or writing a methods section of a paper. Keep these tasks small and specific. Estimate the time it will take—in hours, not days—it will take to do each task. Multiply this time estimate by two. If the task is completed in less time, you will feel wonderful. More likely, unanticipated obstacles will make this seemingly conservative time estimate quite accurate.

If you can delegate the task, and have someone to delegate it to, do it. If you think you can't delegate it, consider hiring or training someone. A task which will take more than ten hours of your time should be subdivided, because it is not specific enough. Seek sub-divisions that permit delegation to others, and budget time for recruiting, training, and supervising them.

The next step is to mesh these tasks into your calendar, realistically allowing for non-research demands on your time. Fill in your calendar in pencil, because unanticipated obstacles will crop up, making revisions essential. Besides, if you don't revise, you won't get the satisfaction of crossing off completed tasks.

Organizational Aids

The structure that you create for yourself on a monthly, weekly, and even daily basis must be made concrete. In particular, you need an appointment book. A simple perusal of any stationery store will reveal wide variety in the kinds of books available. Some books provide for a detailed daily schedule, others provide a week-at-a-glance, and others provide a month-at-a-glance. One of the editors of this volume uses a wall calendar with every day of the year shown! You have to decide which system works for you.

One of the authors uses a month-at-a-glance appointment book. The square for each day is very small (about one-and-a-half inches), and consequently, it is difficult to schedule in very many appointments. Accordingly, plenty of time is left for reading and writing. The month-at-a-glance is then supplemented with a detailed daily schedule.

Some people keep an appointment book only on a day-by-day basis. To our minds, this has two risks. First, one tends to cram too many appointments into a day because there is so much space, and second, it does not give a large view, but rather focuses one's attention on only one day at a time. Consequently, we favor a system that enables one to see the large picture (week, month, or year at a time, depending on one's preference), supplemented with a detailed daily schedule.

Scheduling A Day

You should consciously schedule how you are going to use your time each day. Effective time management begins with an understanding of your circadian rhythms. Each of us has hours when we are at our best and hours when we are fit only for the most mundane tasks. Save your best hours for your high priority research tasks, like writing.

For example, one of the authors divides the day into three sets of four hours. The first four morning hours, beginning at 8:00 a.m., are her best hours. These are inviolably set aside for thinking, writing, and teaching graduate seminars. The next four hours are reserved for moderately demanding tasks, such as teaching undergraduate courses, meeting with research assistants, planning data analyses, and revising papers. The last four hours (and there aren't always four of them) are used for tasks that require little thought: responding to memos, answering letters, writing recommendations, filing, and so forth.

The other author prefers to write for longer periods of time and has the reverse circadian rhythm. On "writing days," her morning starts slowly. She begins by editing the output from her last day of writing, and then moves on to the outline she had prepared for her first half-hour of new writing. By mid-morning, she is thinking or writing at full speed. Afternoons are inviolable: research assistants know not to come by with questions, and all telephone calls are answered by a secretary. Less demanding tasks get done in the evenings and on "non-writing" days.

It obviously does not matter which of these systems you use, or whether you develop one of your own. The point is that, by knowing what your good and bad hours are, you will use your time more efficiently. Moreover, by planning in terms of good and bad hours, you will force yourself to set aside a chunk of time each week for thinking, research, and writing.

Avoid checkerboard days with appointments at 10:00, 12:00, and 3:00, and nothing in between. Try not to organize your schedule around the preferences of others. It is reasonable to ask some other people, particularly students and your research assistants, to accommodate their preferences to yours. You will work far more effectively if you bunch your meetings and appointments together. Each person or event will have to give way to the next, ensuring that meetings which could take twenty minutes don't expand into an hour. Lunches and after-work drinks can serve double duty, as can walks between meeting places. In short, plan your day in detail, so that you get as much done as possible, thus keeping your research time safe from encroachment.

If possible, get a gate-keeper such as a secretary or an R.A. to protect you from interruptions during your thinking and writing time. If you don't have such a person, then develop a hideaway place to do this work. It could be your home, your lab, or a library carrel. Its chief requirements are that it has no phone that must be answered and that people can't find you easily.

As we have implied, the universal pest is the telephone. You need to find a way to escape your telephone regularly. You can sequester yourself in your lab or an office without a phone, or you can get a gate-keeper to let the calls accumulate, as suggested above. Some telephone systems now have call-forwarding, so that your messages can be taken by the main psychology office and you can remain undisturbed. Other people use telephone answering machines. A telephone answering machine may be useful to you if you get a lot of important calls. Neither of the authors does, and consequently, we are more than happy to escape the 10 or so calls we miss by virtue of being away from the phone. To decide if you want to use a telephone answering machine, you might well monitor your calls, determine how many you are getting, figure how badly they are cutting into your work time, and decide whether they are important enough to justify getting the messages. If you decide to use an answering machine, you should indicate clearly when you will return calls or when the caller should plan to call back.

If your days are well-planned and your appointments bunched together, it will be easier to say you are "unfortunately too busy right now" to see some people. Our "too busy" lists include publishers who want to talk about textbooks we have no intention of using or writing, almost all journalists, and anyone who wants to talk about the contents of a paper they have not yet read. Students, however, represent a special kind of demand on your time, which requires separate discussion.

Dealing With Hordes of Students

When you first became an Assistant Professor, you were probably grateful for any student who darkened your door. Now, you probably have more student demands for your time than you, or anyone else, can manage. You must impose limitations on the number and kinds of students you supervise.

In a foolhardy burst of enthusiasm, altruism, and spinelessness, one of the authors spent a year working with nineteen students. The other author, equally spineless, is currently supervising eight doctoral students.

Both numbers are too high, causing nightmares of hordes of students swarming through home and office. When you take on a student, you owe that student a certain amount of time and energy. Every additional student you agree to supervise takes time away from the first. If you take on too many students, you are not doing anyone a favor.

Decide how many students or how many projects you want to cope with simultaneously. Say no when these limits are exceeded. Four (five, tops) graduate students are probably the maximum you can supervise well. To this, you might add four undergraduates only if much of their direct supervision is done by graduate students.

It is hard to avoid being seduced by a bright student with an interesting idea, about which you know little. However, you will have to invest a lot of time learning about this new area, or you will have to trust the student to know the topic thoroughly. All too often, such trust is misplaced, the end-result is unpublishable, and you will have wasted time. Here are some ways to say no that the authors do not utilize frequently enough:

"I am already supervising seven students. Your project sounds very interesting, but I would be doing us both a disservice to agree to supervise it."

"I'm sorry, but I don't serve as a thesis reader when I haven't been involved in the design of the study, as conceptualization and design are the areas where I have found I can be most helpful."

"I'm sorry, but I don't feel I know enough about your subject to be of help. My work is in (give short description that sounds as different from student's topic as possible)."

The Pile

There is a phenomenon known as "the pile," that consists of all the mandatory and discretionary reading which mounts up during the semester or the year. The pile has a life of its own, collapsing, multiplying, and subdividing at irregular intervals. The pile is a sign of poor organization, and it is essential to control it.

The pile is what is left over after you have read and sorted your mail. Thus, the key to controlling the pile lies in how you approach your mail. The first rule is: Never read anything you don't have to. Glance at the sender's name, the title, even the first paragraph or abstract if you have to. Then, make a decision: to read or not to read. Your mail, like anyone's mail, is largely composed of rules and regulations, campus newspapers, changes in policies, many memos, descriptions of books from publishers, and the like. Read the absolute minimum of this material. Much of it will become obsolete on its own. File that which you might someday need and throw the rest away, unread if possible.

The second rule is, with few exceptions: Never read anything twice. Don't read anything until you have to. Circumstances may change, making the reading unnecessary. If you read it too far in advance, you will have to re-read it later. Once you have read something, respond right away. Otherwise, it may be mid-July before you excavate your pile and find it, and by then you will probably have to read it again.

The third rule is: Do not put manuscripts to review in your pile. They will get buried. Three or four months later an editor will write you an angry letter asking whether you intend to review a particular paper. If you intend to it, do so quickly. If you do not intend to review it, return it immediately with a plausible reason.

If you have followed these guidelines, then your pile should be composed virtually entirely of papers you might want to read. Even this pile can and should be drastically shrunk. By "chronologizing," you can gear your reading to your teaching and research. For example, if an interesting paper on self-schemas comes in your mail, save it for the week you are teaching this topic in your graduate seminar. Put it in the file for that week of the course. When the time comes to prepare for that class, that file will contain papers which you can use to fill out your lectures. Simultaneously, you will be keeping on top of the literature in this area. A similar approach can be used with papers germane to your research. Keep a file of work relevant to each of your projects, and read through the abstracts, and perhaps the papers, before you start designing or writing.

Chronologizing will reduce your pile of papers to those which you have no immediate purpose for reading. Throw many of these away too. Select a few to file, in case you need them in the future. Don't save too many, as it is amazing how quickly you can fill ten file cabinets. The only thing left in your pile should be four or five "gems," that is, papers which have been written by people who consistently make strong contributions to the field. If you are an inveterate reader, you might want to add one or two "flyers" which have captured your imagination. You can give yourself these for dessert someday, after a particularly productive bout of writing.

Getting Time to Rest and Gain Perspective

The rhythm of the academic year provides natural opportunities for you to rest, think, evaluate your work, and change your course of action if you so desire. A few weeks before a new semester or quarter begins and the summer before a fall are good times to reevaluate one's activities and the use of one's time. Remember the research on incubation effects, which demonstrates that solutions to problems often crop up at unlikely moments when the mind is seemingly at rest, but actually liberated to solve a problem on its own. Free times, including extended free time during summers and sabbaticals, can provide you with this opportunity.

To take full advantage of these times may require your getting away. In the summer, for example, it is useful to take some of that time off. When you come back to your work, you may find that your priorities have changed, and trivial tasks that seemed so important when you left have faded into their rightful importance. If you are fortunate enough to get a sabbatical semester or even a year, try to take it away from your university. For some, particularly those involved in dual-career relationships, this may be difficult to do. However, if you stay at your home university, you will be tempted to work with just a few students, or do just a few administrative favors for the chairperson in your department, and soon you will discover that your sabbatical has been eroded by precisely the dross you were trying to avoid.

There are several criteria for picking a sabbatical location. Try to pick a host institution that will not make formal demands on your time, but that will provide you with office space and one or more stimulating colleagues in your area. It would help if the university were located in a setting with exciting cultural opportunities and good food and wine. Provence, we hear, is lovely in the spring. The London theater is breathtaking in winter. In short, the sabbatical time is a time when you can reward yourself for all the hard work you have done while simultaneously stimulating your mind in preparation for the work that is to come.

LIFE OUTSIDE OF WORK

Yes, there is, or there should be, life outside of work. It is, however, probably not an accident that this section of the paper is shorter than the preceding two. The stressful first years eat up your energy and hitting your stride almost always means regular, long hours of work. Despite the fact that it is hard to find room for it, the rest of your life is critical. After all, why are you working so hard and using your work time so efficiently, if not to enjoy your private life and your work?

A strong private life can be an insurance policy. At some time your work life, like everyone else's, will temporarily collapse around your ears. A grant proposal that you were counting on may not come through. An article which is particularly important to you may be rejected. When these things happen, and they certainly will, it helps to have the rest of your life to fall back on.

Your work life and your personal life exist in an uneasy symbiosis. What happens in one arena affects the other. If you devote too much time to your work, your work as well as your private life may suffer. Studies suggest that workaholics may get more work done, but the work is generally of lower quality than that produced by people who work at a more sensible pace. Workaholics can spend endless time subdividing the pile or perfecting the perfect coding system. The rest of your life should not solely be designed to make your work life go more smoothly. However, if the rest of your life is in balance, your work will go better too.

Your Personal Life

Your private life is private and you know best what you need to thrive. Undoubtedly, our parents and teachers were right when they urged us to eat well, exercise, sleep sometimes, and have a social life. The latter is particularly important, as social support is essential, in order to cope successfully with the tension and time pressure of this strange career we have chosen. Many people find the most important source of support to be family and friends. You should spend time with them now, or they won't be there when you need them. Schedule time for your leisure life, or it may go by the board in a crunch. Buy concert tickets in advance, so you'll have to go. Set up a regular tennis game. Have a regular bi-weekly dinner with a group of friends. Children offer personal rewards and have special needs for parents' presence, and so merit separate treatment below.

Starting a Family

No sane person would ever try to combine a family and career without a wife-equivalent, if he or she fully understood what it entailed. Balancing a demanding career and parenthood is a logistical nightmare. Inevitably, children take time away from work and vice-versa. Yet, few who have started families regret the decision. This is more than simply post-decisional rationalization. Children add a particular dimension to life that seems to be unobtainable in other ways: thrilling, joyous, and playful.

As is already clear, this section of the chapter, even more than the rest, reflects our personal experiences. Your opinions may well differ. These are arenas where people, both reasonable and unreasonable, have a long history of disagreement.

We have chosen to direct our remarks to women, although we hope that male readers may also be interested. We made this choice because women bear the brunt of the problems associated with pregnancy and childbirth. In addition, time studies indicate that female professionals with full-time jobs cope with more than half, generally much more than half, of the child care and housekeeping tasks as well. Thus, particularly if you are a female, balancing a career and a family may well take a toll on your vita. Few who look at your reduced output will regard your family as a legitimate reason for it.

Some say there is a right time to start a family. This is a myth. There are pros and cons associated with any period of your career. In some ways, having children as a doctoral student is the easiest, providing there is a supportive environment. This might include a partner willing to do a good part of the work, relatives willing to take care of the baby, or inexpensive, high-quality day care. You will never again have as much time as when you are a doctoral student, a fact which should be clear by this point in the chapter. You are younger and have more energy now than you will have later, no matter how much your thesis has exhausted you.

Having a child during your pre-tenure years also has advantages. You are still fairly young, so risks in childbirth are lessened. Moreover, you have greater financial resources than in graduate school, making it easier to pay for child care and household help. The disadvantage, of course, is the pressure of the tenure crunch.

The greatest advantage of starting a family after tenure is just that: it is post-tenure. However, by waiting so long, you run the risk of having difficulty getting pregnant, and the birth will be more risky to both the child and the mother. Furthermore, you will probably have lost some of the energy you had in your twenties, making it difficult to cope with the simultaneous demands of a full and active career and an active family. By this time you may also have taken on enough formal obligations, such as chairing your department, that it may be difficult to get the time you will need to give your family.

There are other alternatives: interrupting your career or drastically slowing it down, for example, by working part-time. If you choose these options, it is best to do it very early or after you are well settled. In any case, you should know that, given the current structure of academic life, interrupting or slowing your career will have costs. It will be difficult to pick up where you left off. After several years, the literature will have changed, there will be new data analysis techniques, and the start-up and catching-up process will be a time-consuming handicap. Tilly Olsen's words capture the dilemma eloquently: "It is distraction, not meditation, that becomes habitual; interruption, not continuity; spasmodic, not constant, toil. Work interrupted, deferred, postponed makes blockage—at best, less accomplishment. Unused capacities atrophy, cease to be"

(1978, p. 33). These problems can be overcome with great effort, but the handicap is real.

Regardless of the timing of your family, if you continue working, you will be under some scrutiny by your colleagues. Some may doubt that you are spending enough time on your career. Consequently, it is useful to try to determine what stereotypes these scrutinizers may hold and do specific things that indicate their inaccuracy. One thing that you should do is make yourself visible when you are in the department.

One of the authors coped with the responsibilities of a job and small children by delegating everything possible to her secretary. The secretary picked up mail, ran errands, xeroxed papers, discussed personnel matters, handled the business matters on the grant, and did all of the other things that the author occasionally did for herself. The consequence of what seemed to be an intelligent use of time was that a substantial number of her colleagues thought she was never coming into the office! Once this became apparent, she made sure to go to the faculty mailroom to collect her mail at a time when most of the other faculty members did the same to signal clearly that she was working. In addition, staying after normal working hours for an occasional meeting, although inconvenient, is probably worth it for what it signals. Likewise, this is probably not a time to miss most faculty meetings. On the other hand, one should not go too far in the other direction. In order to carry out the dual role successfully, you will need time to think and write. The time you have in the office is very precious and you do not want to clutter it up with B+ tasks.

Ironically, some of your scrutinizers may be concerned that you are not spending enough time with your babies. For this group of people, it may be important to show that you are concerned as a mother, that you have the same problems, conflicts, and lack of sleep that they had when they were young. Do talk about your children with your colleagues. Many of them will be interested. Most of them have had children, and there is no reason why you can't as well.

The difficulties of combining a career and a family do not have easy solutions. A few possibilities, that we or our acquaintances have found useful, include the following. One way of coping with the load is to find a way to buy some time off. Some people have done this by securing a fellowship or grant which enables them to work on a more flexible schedule, freeing them from committee work and some teaching. In this way, their commitment to high-quality research and writing is sustained, whereas some of the time-consuming, less important tasks are eliminated.

The way you organize your time may also change. Typically, poorly organized people find that they have to get better organized, and well-organized people become positively breathtaking in the perfection of their systems. One's every waking moment is used efficiently. Letters of recommendation are written during colloquia, the next day's schedule is planned during faculty meetings, and lunch is combined with a meeting. Home life, too, becomes more organized. Shopping, laundry, and errands go on as firm a schedule as writing.

Perhaps the most important aid in combining a family with a career is to have a system that reliably and regularly frees one for work, with a back-up system in case the regular system fails. The regular system might be organized daycare or a person who comes to your house. Back-up systems might include friends who also have children. You will need someone you can depend on that awful day when you have to chair an oral defense of a thesis, and the daycare center has closed down because the sewers have broken down.

Trying to combine careers with a family can also take an inadvertent toll on one's relationship with one's spouse. Tasks around the house often take on a zero-sum character: if you don't do it, then the other person must, and the sheer number of tasks with one or more children is astonishing. A full-time chauffeur would make only a dent.

Inevitably, this creates problems for professional opportunities. Being invited to give a colloquium at a major university far from your home means that the spouse must pick up all of the work while you are gone. Even attending a convention becomes a major I.O.U. situation. A professional advancement for one person may bring pleasures, increased financial resources, and increased time commitments, and consequently, the other spouse may have to fill the breach. Emotional strains can result.

There are no easy solutions to this problem, but a few things help. First, it helps to keep clearly in mind why these problems have been created: there is simply too much to do, and no one is particularly at fault. Second, it is useful to delegate as many of the joint tasks to other people as possible. A cleaning person a couple of times a week, a once-a-week gardener if necessary and affordable, or a regularly scheduled babysitter to create an occasional couple of hours, can go a long way. Many dual-career couples with children schedule regular times to get together just to talk. One couple we know has dinner together every Saturday night, with a rule that neither one of them can talk about what clever things the children have done this week.

There are inevitable casualties of these herculean efforts at a dual life. Quiet drinks with colleagues are rare, and spontaneous dinners with friends, unless they too have children, shrink to a minimum. Getting an extra two or three hours in the evening to finish a project in time for a deadline inevitably means a trade in time later. Personally, we have found the sacrifices worth it, without question.

The Pleasures of Working

Private life is obviously not the only source of pleasure open to you. Most of us chose to be professors because we thought we would enjoy the work, perhaps the satisfactions of research, the relationships to students, the process of teaching, the excuse for continuing to learn, or the freedom to decide what we want to study. In this chapter, we have discussed primarily the demands, rather than the joys, of academic life. The joys, however, are the primary reasons why this stressful, ill-paid line of work is worth pursuing. Personally, what drives us ultimately is the pure joy of science: "Those moments . . . when suddenly there is a synthesis of the human intelligence . . . and to know every day that it might happen again" (Gornick, 1983, p.52).

If you enjoy your work, the pleasures of the process will be evident to you. However, there may be some minor advantages and pleasures of your job that you may have overlooked. For example, as a faculty member your time is flexible. Yet, many professors treat their positions as nine-to-five jobs. As long as you work enough hours, why hold yourself to a rigid schedule that may not be conducive to other needs in your life? If your writing is going well, why not write until dawn and sleep some other time? If it is not going well, why not go have some fun?

Academia also gives you the flexibility to choose where you work. You do not have to be in your office all the time. If you are so inclined, you can sit outside and write; you can work at home or in a library. You also have some flexibility in the tasks that you do. On one hand, you do not want to develop work habits that are positively weird in the context of your colleagues, but on the other hand, some deviation is clearly acceptable. Unlike most jobs, a faculty position also gives you considerable discretion in choosing what problems you want to study and what tasks you want to do next. If you have been writing a paper, and the words are not coming, then turn to something else. Make hedonistic decisions about what you are working on. If you always do what you think you are supposed to be doing, and never try out something that you think might be unexpectedly absorbing, then you will ultimately feel robbed. Moreover, you cannot blame your job for robbing you. You have robbed yourself.

Another perk is the occasional conference to which you will be invited. As an Assistant Professor, of course, your first conferences may be in factory towns with no social or cultural attractions. Cheer up. Eventually, you will be invited to better places, and when you are, this will give you an opportunity to explore an exciting new city. Make sure you take the time to do so.

This hedonistic approach to work is important to us. It explains why we work so hard to manage our time and it explains why, from time to time, we abandon our rational plans and do exactly what we feel we would enjoy—like writing this chapter.

REFERENCES

Gornick, V. (August 1983). Women in science. *Savvy. 4,* 44–52.
Lakein, A. (1973). *How to get control of your time and your life.* New York: Signet.
Mackenzie. R. A. (1972). *The time trap: Managing your way out.* New York: AMACON.
Olsen, T. (1978). *Silences.* New York: Delacorte Press.

---

[1]Editors' note: It is to be hoped that the authors' "extra" advice to beginning female and minority faculty members will be heeded by those of us who are more senior, sensitizing us to our prejudices and stereotypes. Perhaps, then, such advice will become dated!

3

POWER AND POLITICS IN ACADEMIC DEPARTMENTS

Gerald R. Salancik
Carnegie-Mellon University

Attitudes about power in academic institutions slip easily from disgust to awe. Some scientists resent its presence. Others deny it has anything to do with them. A few chase after it with sniggering glee. Most people just accept its part in their lives and use or ignore it as they need.

Whatever your attitude, one thing to be clear about is that power exists in every institution affecting you. It is in the department employing you; the granting agencies subsidizing your research; the journals publishing you. As long as you want something and it conflicts with what others want, power emerges, if it doesn't already exist, to determine who will get what. For you, this may be a workable teaching schedule, or travel money or enough computer time. Or it may be a grant, and the relevant power may not be yours but your institution's.

This chapter attempts to give you some of the knowledge you may need for coping with power in the organizations of psychology. We describe how power arises and is used. The aim is to paint a picture of academic power that we hope will help you understand the world you are entering. This description summarizes numerous studies that colleagues (Jeffrey Pfeffer, Huseyin Leblebici, Barry Staw) and I have done in past years—studies of universities, granting agencies, academic departments, departmental administrators, committees, scientific disciplines, and journals. It also lays the foundation for our second task, which is to offer some guidelines about building your bases of influence and using them sensibly and effectively. We call on personal experiences and the experiences of our friends, though, admittedly, none of us were particularly adept in dealing with the political realities we faced when we started as assistant professors.

Maybe your start will be easier. Having been a graduate student you probably know a lot about power already. You hustled resources like typewriters or paper from departmental staff, probably traded your expertise for the expertise of colleagues in other areas, bargained for fellowships or just managed the conflicting demands of your faculty to buy yourself time to study. Some of your mates you might remember as getting better deals on their research assignments because they were aligned with major figures in the department. And you probably know colleagues whose first jobs came because their faculty were well connected.

After graduate school, you'll find the need to hustle for small favors abates. But other political considerations take its place. You still need other people and resources. You need libraries, computers, software, textbooks, experimental subjects, laboratory equipment, writing materials, mailing and telephone services, to name but a few of the material resources psychologists consume in great quantities. But you need less tangible things also. There's the peace of mind you need to concentrate; the cooperation you need to access research sites; the political freedom you need to dissect your laboratory animals or interview your human subjects; the autonomy you need to schedule your time to think or read. And then there are the endless gifts and favors that you need. These come from the colleagues who listen to your views or read your papers; the students who take down your words; the administrators who smile obliquely with encouragement; the audiences that attend your colloquia; the lovers and companions who offer you warmth and security. The list goes on. And the more you want to get done, the longer your list of dependencies.

Having been a graduate student, you also probably appreciate that these resources are too scarce to satisfy all the legitimate demand for them. They are things everybody wants and only some can have. Unless you control their allocation, you easily deduce that much depends on decisions of other people. Our mentors, our colleagues, our secretaries, department heads, granting agencies, even the subjects in our experiments, make these decisions. In deciding, they affect how we do our work, whether we get the resources we need, whether we keep our work loads to manageable and satisfactory levels, whether we complete a study, whether we get a paper written up for publication or, even, a written paper typed.

As a professor, then, you'll face many political needs. What do you do? How do you put yourself in a position to get what you need without hassle? Without indignity? How do you even learn about the power that affects you? How much emphasis should you put on politics or how do you handle yourself in a department of more experienced political actors? Should you "play politics"? Or avoid them? Should you align yourself with powerful interests in the department and in your discipline? Or should you keep to yourself, conducting your own affairs, doing your work, publishing your research? Should you become involved in the politics of the university?

In the pages that follow we try to provide the knowledge that will help you decide your answers to these questions. There are no rigid rules, because the answers will depend on your situation, on what you want and on the systemic nature of power in that situation. The place to start is with a clear picture of what power is and how it is used.

WHERE IS THE POWER ANYWAY?

What is known about organizational power can be stated very succinctly. Power exists in all organizations and is essential to their operation. It arises from the dependencies that individuals and groups in the organiztion have for one another and it concentrates in ways that resolve conflicts in favor of the most critical dependencies. These most critical dependencies themselves originate from an organization's environment and its relations with other organizations. You would do well to understand these three points, for they will help you to put yourself in situations that serve your interests rather than oppose them.

Consider the case of a colleague at another university. We call her Janet. Janet was 5 years out of graduate school. When she finished her degree, the job market was, shall we say, soft. Janet was more fortunate than many of her friends, though, and got a job at one of the better schools, the only woman psychologist hired in its 60 odd years. Perhaps because she appreciated her fortune, Janet didn't worry much about the details of the offer when she accepted it. Two details she should have been concerned about were the department's provision for summer salary and convention travel money. Both, it later turned out, were available and both were critical to Janet's future.

Janet built up a fair-sized debt in school. When she neared the end of her first year, she asked about summer support so she could devote herself to research. The department head, leaning back in his chair, told her the department had committed its summer research budget already and had assumed she did not need any because she hadn't said so when she was hired. "But," said the head, "if you want to teach, we could at least get that for you." Janet took the teaching offer and, of course, aborted much of the research she had planned.

The next few years saw similar exchanges. Each time there was some reason Janet couldn't get what she needed. Her most recent "surprise" came when she sought funds to go to a special conference in her research area. Again she went to her department head. He explained that the department's travel policy was to cover the complete expenses of one trip per year per faculty member and that she could choose any conference she wanted to attend in the United States. "Well," Janet interrupted, "I would like to go to APA this year, since I'm going to present a paper. But I'd also need to go to this special conference, as it's very important for my work." Again, the department head told her the policy and pointed out that while he normally had some discretionary funds, they were committed already. "I wish I had known this earlier," he said as Janet left.

Janet was quickly behind in her work relative to colleagues who had entered the department with her. And comparisons between her and her colleagues were never more than a whisper away, whispers she heard clearly enough to realize she might not be promoted with them.

Power Concentrates Around Critical Dependencies

Janet's problems arose from her department's very ordinary politics. Where is the power in this situation? The department head? Let's explore what makes the department head powerful. First is the fact that Janet, like others in her department, wants a particular resource. Second, neither Janet nor the others have what they want. Third, the department head temporarily controls its allocation, with discretion to dispense it any way he wishes. These conditions are necessary and sufficient for the creation of the department head's power. You want something and somebody else has the freedom and capability to provide it that you lack. If any of these were not true, there would be no power. If Janet and the others cared not a hoot for summer and travel monies, the head would reign over an empty realm. If these funds were nondiscretionary and had to be allotted according to some incontrovertible standards, the head would be reduced to a keeper of books, tallying requests and dispersing funds.

In short, the department head is powerful because of the role his position plays in the department. Power concentrates into his position precisely to resolve conflicts of the kind embroiling Janet. Departments are not the same in this regard. Some don't concentrate power as much, and permit their heads little say. In my university, there are two types of departmental administrators. One is called a head; the other a chair. The choice of words is probably not accidental. A head is a lifetime position. Its occupant authorizes all departmental educational, budget, hiring, promotion, and salary decisions. It is a very powerful position and much like headships at other universities. The chair position, in contrast, is temporary. Its resident is obligated to attend to the advice of the elected "executive committee" of a department. This position doesn't concentrate power in the administrator but leaves it with the faculty.

How much power concentrates into organizational positions—chairs, heads, deans, grant administrators, committees—will depend on the extent of an organization's conflicting interests. The chair administrative form we described, for instance, arises when faculty are unable to resolve their conflicts into directions that all interests will support. Through an elective process, the contestants ensure their points of view will be represented in the executive committee where they can bargain and negotiate with one another. Often they shuffle back and forth between positions because no group is able to convince the others of its greater merit. This form arises in fields with less agreed-upon paradigms. It's more common in the social sciences; more rare in the physical sciences.

When power concentrates into formal positions as it does in most academic departments, the concentration serves the needs of dominant interests in a department. A head can move a department in particular directions with vigor, neglecting some interests at one point in time and others at another. A department head, however, cannot long get away with consistently neglecting major interests in the department. Anyone who has seen a department head roll when it displeases critical faculty knows how trepidatious tenancy can be.

Power in a department, then, rests with a department's faculty, or at least some of them. Where then was the power in Janet's situation? To find out, Janet talked to associates about what else was going on in the department and who was getting the funds she needed.

The story quickly got sorted out. The department had been building its cognitive psychology group for the past few years and the monies that Janet wasn't getting were going to newer faculty in these areas and, in some cases, older faculty. This happened with enough frequency on enough issues that a reasonable statistician would conclude it was not random.

At first Janet got annoyed and wondered if she was being discriminated against as a woman. Later she thought about why the department head was leaning toward the cognitive group just then. The group was growing; its faculty were building a graduate program and were starting to fund it with a few large grants. The departmental budget had barely been keeping pace and, although the overall doctoral program had grown slightly, government cutbacks hurt the social, clinical, and experimental groups severely in the last two years.

Annoyance drifted to depression as Janet realized that what was going on was more systematic than a few unlucky lost opportunities. Although the head was powerful, his power only mirrored the faculty's. Yet it seemed all faculty were not equal. The cognitive group, as Orwell would have it, were more equal. Decisions reflected their interests the most. Why? Because the doctoral program of the rest of the department depended on the cognitive group's larger coffers.

Although the details in other departments may differ from those in

Janet's, the general situation is typical. Power organizes around those subgroups (departments, disciplinary groups, or individuals) in an organization thought to contribute its most critical resources.

The External Basis for Organizational Power

Janet's situation shows us organizational power is not a personal quality of the fortunate or greedy. It is situational. The cognitive faculty were powerful not because of any particularly charming qualities they possessed. They were powerful because they contributed what the department needed just then. This role was more circumstantial than deliberate. It followed a few unfavorable decisions of U.S. presidents and a developing industry in computer intelligence.

Ultimately, power in academic institutions originates outside them. We can see this easily in the growth of the physical sciences following John Kennedy's decision to go to the moon, and in the growth and decline of the social sciences following Lyndon Johnson's decision to end poverty and Ronald Reagan's decision to begin it again. We can see this also in our own universities. Departments in universities, and the areas within them, represent different disciplines, each somewhat separate from the others. Each discipline has its own sources of funding, its own markets for faculty and students, its own journals, and its own definitions and markets for prestige. Although some intellectual strands link them, and although they compete at some level for funds, students, and public attention, disciplines for the most part operate independently. These facts form the bases for the distribution of power in universities and departments.

Departments are rarely equal in their power. Some command larger shares of resources, have an easier time getting their people hired and promoted, have lighter teaching loads or more teaching assistance distributed to them. Different groups dominate in different universities. Prestigious private universities are more likely than prestigious public universities to have outstanding law and business schools, and prestigious public universities are more likely to have outstanding engineering and agricultural schools. These differences reflect the historical flow of resources into the institutions. In a similar way, the distribution of power among and within departments results from the way resources come into them and the roles they play.

Grants and Power in a University

In my former university, The University of Illinois, the most powerful departments come from the physical sciences. It doesn't take much to see this. Most of the important committees in the university are peopled by faculty from the physics, mathematics, and engineering departments. The only well-represented behavioral science department is psychology. Curious about the dominance of these groups, a colleague and I studied 13 years of the university's history, examining the budgets, grants, teaching loads, academic rankings (ACE ratings), and such, of more than half of the departments in the university. The departments on key committees were allotted larger portions of the state budget relative to other departments and disproportionate to their teaching obligations to undergraduate or graduate students. The budget of one physical science department, for instance, correlated .73 with its 13-year growth in its undergraduate teaching, whereas a comparable correlation for one social science department was −.64. Allocations to the powerful were also disproportionate to their academic rankings, despite frequent claims that the limited funds of the university should go to the "better" departments. In these 13 years, a top-ranked psychology department was not quite worth as much as a top-ranked electrical engineering department.

It is not difficult to figure out what was accounting for the budget decisions. One need remember only that power distributes along the lines of critical dependencies. The University of Illinois is a major research institution. Research and graduate education are its primary goals. Talk about them invades every meeting and colors every issue requiring organizational attention. Recognizing this, it was easy to deduce that the most critical contributions the departments made to the university were the resources needed to run large-scale graduate programs. These didn't come from the State of Illinois in the amounts required, either. They came from grants.

Grants are important in universities for two reasons. The less important reason is that they fund research. This, however nice for faculty and students, benefits mainly the department getting the grant, not the university as a whole. Grants would not be a basis for power in a university if that were all they did. The second, and more important, role of grants is that they contribute discretionary monies in the form of overhead rebates.

Shared between the campus administration and the departments generating them, overhead funds play a key role in maintaining quality in educational and research programs throughout a university. They accumulate into piles of money available for activities unjustified by other budgetary categories. Their greatest value is that they are discretionary. They benefit research by providing seed money to projects awaiting grant support or groundwork for frontier areas that haven't attracted government or foundation attention yet. They benefit teaching by funding innovations beyond the reach of the normal educational budget. Without them, the developments in computer learning would have advanced little.

Discretionary funds also play a big role in managing a university. They can be critical in attracting and keeping talented faculty and students. A smart department head can promise the wavering support for special projects or summer research, competing more effectively than without such funds. And when the discretionary funds in one department are used up, a head in good standing with campus administrators can petition to dip into their much larger discretionary piles. The University of Illinois recently amassed a million dollar funding and equipment package to attract the inventor of magnetic resonance imaging. Fifteen campus units cooperated and much of the support came from discretionary monies.

With grants generating such critical discretionary funds, it wasn't surprising to find a department's power was proportional to its contributions to the overhead pool. The major predictor of the differences between the power of departments was the grant monies they provided. Seventy percent of the variance in power measures was associated with contract funds, and power in turn was the major predictor of state budget allocations. What this meant is that the small fractional discretionary funds provided by some departments promoted their control of the rest of the budget. With only slight hyperbole, 10% of the resources determined how 80% of the budget was spent!

One cannot simply extrapolate these results to other institutions. Universities differ in their goals, and more important, in the factors affecting their survival. For the University of Illinois, the quality of its graduate and research programs is very important, and not an easy task given the constraints of its environment.

Other universities organize around other resources. The one generality is that power plays a role in every university and derives from the critical resources that shape that institution's success and ultimately its survival. Private schools, lacking the subsidies of a state appropriation process, operate very differently than public universities. They survive by accumulating endowment, which depends on their graduates' wealth and willingness to part with it as they age. Not surprisingly, private schools pay a lot more attention to their undergraduates' experiences. They want their students to leave with warm feelings and fond memories. And this affects their decisions as much as grants do at the University of Illinois. It just affects them in different ways.

POWER IN USE

A discussion of power would not be very useful if it either had no effect on decisions or its effects were ubiquitous. In the first case, it would be irrelevant to us and, in the second, it would be superfluous. Power in academic institutions is neither of these. In this section we describe what is known about the conditions under which power is used. It is not used to resolve every conflict, and the conflicts it resolves are usually those unresolved by other means.

People enter into political activity under rather specific conditions, mainly when the resources involved are critical to their own purposes and when the resources are scarce, when more seek them than can have them. Sensible people don't waste time debating issues that are either unimportant or assured. But even when resources are scarce and needed, faculty may not be inclined to pursue them with unrelenting political tenacity. Quite often we simply agree with one another about the legitimacy of claims on resources. If two of our colleagues want to attend APA at a time when the travel budget is too lean to support both, the department head might simply tell one, "I've discussed this with the executive committee and we've agreed to give preference to younger faculty and faculty presenting papers." This is a familiar enough statement, and the disadvantaged faculty member would likely accept it without feeling outraged or slighted. Few would construe the policy as very political.

The Role of Social Uncertainty

Power most visibly affects decisions when there is a lack of agreement about what should be done or how to do it. The brutal truth of this principle was made very clear to me from a story my brother related about Viet Nam. My retelling is stylized, but the essentials are true. There were three soldiers in a medical tent, a corporal, a lieutenant, and a medical officer. The corporal and lieutenant both needed blood according to the medical officer. Unfortunately, there was only enough blood for one man. Societies have evolved two principles to solve allocation problems like this. One is said to be the principle of socialism—to each according to his need. The other is said to be the principle of capitalism—to each according to his worth. The principle of need is obviously unable to resolve true problems of scarce resource when many are judged needy. The principle of value is more generally applicable, though it requires Solomonic judgment to apply. Is a corporal more worthy than a lieutenant because he can kill many enemy? Or is a lieutenant more valuable because he can lead many corporals into battle? The army has no difficulty with this question. A person of rank is automatically to be considered more valuable. The legitimacy of this rule, however, was not as apparent to the corporal as it was to the officers who wrote it. He simply picked up a rifle, pointed it at the captain, and said, "You or him, doc." This is the principle of power. It quickly sorts out what people consider valuable. The doctor, like the corporal, thought his own life was more important than the lieutenant's.

Grants and Power Between Universities

Allocations based on rules of need and worth then are useful up to the point of disagreement. When people disagree, social and political factors seem to play a larger role in decision making. My colleagues and I observed this in the allocations of the National Science Foundation. We studied grants made during an 8-year period to departments from four social sciences—economics, psychology, sociology, and political science.

Disciplines differ in the extent to which they share ideas about the needs and proper ways of studying phenomena. The four social sciences mentioned above, for instance, are ordered according to the extent of their agreement. Thomas Kuhn called such differences paradigm differences. Physics, in this sense, was said to have a "well-developed" paradigm and sociology, a "less-developed" paradigm. Social psychologists might say fields display more or less of a consensus about research priorities and proprieties. A group of physicists on a grant panel might read a particular work, look at one another and say "Well, that's pretty bad, isn't it?" and move quickly on to the next. Since they share fairly much the same ideas about what research is needed and how it should be done, it is easy to determine if a proposal is up to snuff. Now consider some sociologists facing the same difficult task. One hears a quite different conversation, "Well, on the one hand. . . . But on the other . . ." Or, "Hmmm, this is a bit out of my area. . . . What do you think?"

My colleagues and I reasoned from this, and from principles of Leon Festinger's social comparison theory, that social and political factors would affect decisions more in fields with less developed paradigms. Using both cross-sectional and time-lagged analyses of NSF grants dispersed to departments within economics, psychology, sociology, and political science, we studied historical relations between the amounts allotted departments, the national rankings of departments, and the size of departments, and also whether departments had members on the granting panels. We expected that departments' panel memberships in any year would predict grant allocations to departments in that year more for the fields with less developed paradigms, after controlling for size, rank, and past allocations.

Such indeed was the case. In all disciplines, departments received more grants when they were represented on NSF panels. But in political science and sociology, representation on review panels was substantially more important for predicting grants than departmental ranking or size. Similar observations characterize other grant programs, hiring practices, and journal editorial board appointments. Our interpretation is that when there is less consensus about the merits of people or their work, decision makers must rely on social information to a greater extent.

Paradigm differences can play an equally important role within universities. Departments from disciplines with less consensus experience more conflict in their departmental affairs when resources are scarce. Research indicates they are more likely, for instance, to turn over their department heads. Psychology departments with large paradigm differences among its subareas might witness similar turmoil. As a colleague suggested, "One occasionally notices a physiologist who seems to believe that if it isn't physiological it isn't science." One probably also notices a clinical psychologist or two wondering if the physiologists should keep their brain samples in biology departments and leave psychology to people interested in minds not chemicals. Such stereotypes may just be innocent jostling or they may cover up more deep-seated conflicts of interest in departments. The innocent bystanding new professor can avoid a lot of grief by making contacts across subareas, finding out what their faculty do and, perhaps more important, reminding them of the scientific rigors they all share.

Political effects of intellectual mismatches also show up at the campus level when decisions are taken by groups composed of researchers from numerous fields of knowledge. A typical solution to difficulties of communicating across disciplines when evaluating the quality of a promotion candidate's work is to defer to people within the discipline. From the point of view of the candidate, it is thus very important that there be individuals on the university tenure committee who represent his or her discipline, people who can translate the candidate's discipline to the members of the tenure committee who do not share the assumptions of that discipline. A prudent department head, moreover, should time a person's promotion to fit the composition of a committee. And if a department head is not prudent, a promotion candidate should try to advance or defer the review. Most universities allow a 1- or 2-year leeway on the review process.

The issue here is a very simple one. If evaluators do not share the scientific paradigm of a candidate, no matter how smart and well-intentioned they might be, they will have a difficult time evaluating the candidate. This difficulty also leads universities, granting agencies, and journals to rely heavily on external evaluations. Unable to determine the value of something themselves, they defer to those they believe can. This leads to social and political considerations playing a large role in the decisions that affect scientists. Journal editors and major researchers are asked more frequently than others to make evaluations about members of their discipline. The reason for this probably has less to do with their unique abilities to review than the political needs of a department chair to create information that will be considered credible by others in their institutions. Stanford has a reputation for calling up the "top" people in a discipline when they are considering somebody for a promotion. If these individuals are willing to state that the candidate is a "top" scholar in the area, then the person is given tenure, or so the reputation goes. One suspects this is as much an image-making device for Stanford as a selection device. Through it they get the "top" people in a discipline to admit that Stanford also has the "top" people in its departments. In the end it would appear there would be so many tops in one field that there would not be enough other heads left in the field to spin in admiration.

Yet, such practices do affect decisions, and from the point of view of those who are affected, particularly in fields with less developed paradigms, the use of social bases for decision making implies that members of those fields cannot afford to ignore their social relationships. Going to meetings, letting people know who you are, being introduced by individuals who are already accepted in the field—all of these become critical activities.

MANAGING YOUR OWN POLITICAL SITUATION

A good place to start in considering your political position is to assess your dependencies and the dependencies of others on you. Through them your power and theirs arise. Your goal here should be to minimize your dependencies as much as you can and still fulfill your goals. You want to be in a position to accomplish what you want, whatever its domain—personal, professional, or civic. To do this, you're going to need as much freedom and control as you can muster. And getting it will not be easy when your obligations expand as rapidly as they do in a new job. Mastering your workload, getting organized, setting priorities, using time well—all of these are essential.

Recognizing Your Dependencies

Your discretion is your most valuable resource. If you give it up easily, you'll end up pursuing other people's purposes rather than your own. If you need a lot from other people to accomplish what you want, then they, not you, control your fate. The more things you can do within your own resources, the better off you are. Your own resources are just that—yours. You can do with them as you wish.

It is probably useful to get into the habit of distinguishing the things you can do on your own from the things you require of others. You can write a paper on your own if you have paper and pencil. You can't publish one on your own. You can do some types of research on your own, such as proving theorems. Others you can't, such as surveying a national probability sample. In getting control of your dependencies, you need to know who you must rely on to accomplish your goals. This includes friends, spouses, and children. If you are responsible for a small child and want to write a book, you need blocks of time free from the child. That means you will need to allocate care of the child to someone else. This person becomes someone you depend on, simultaneously a resource and a constraint.

The next step in controlling your dependencies is to reduce them to those that serve your "real" interests. This can be difficult. It requires assessing very realistically three things—how much you really want something, how easy it is to get the resources you need for it, and how much discretion you lose in getting the resources. Planning what to do forces a simultaneous choice of deciding what you really want and whether the cost (in discretion) is really worth the result. Many things you start out thinking you want quickly lose their intrigue when they cost you so much in your freedom that getting them prevents you from getting other things you want. When people say, "Set your priorities!" this is what they mean.

The difficulty in setting priorities is that our desires conflict with one another. We saw this in Janet's situation. Her wish to pay off her debt pressed her into teaching her first summer, taking time away from the other things she wanted. She also wanted to develop a reputation in her discipline area as a major contributor to its research agenda. Her hope that first summer was to generate data she needed for a grant proposal. If she had gotten the grant, her subsequent need for travel money would have abated. Without it, she ended up relying on her department head.

Janet is no different from any of us. We all want conflicting things. Depending on how we choose which ones to emphasize at particular times, we bind ourselves to one set of dependencies or another. The importance of planning is to be sure that the dependencies you are accepting serve your interests. To the greatest extent possible, one tries to keep dependencies to those that can be relied upon.

Recognizing Your Importance in Your Organizations

In Janet's case, she might have thought she could rely on the department head. But it became obvious over time that the department head was preoccupied with other interests. Whether you get the resources you require from others may depend quite often on your importance to them. It's for this reason you want to try to choose your dependencies very carefully.

Ideally, if you rely on others, you want them to be people who will consider your interests in their decision making. Easy enough to say; but how do you get yourself in this position? A good start is to assess seriously what your position is in the organizations that affect you. If you are already in an advantaged position, then you probably need to do little more than maintain it. If not, then you need to enhance your value by contributing to their interests. We address these in turn.

Assessing your political position is a matter of answering a few simple questions about your place and the place of your unit in the larger scheme of things. Although you are probably not likely to have interest or need to get involved in the politics of your university—or even your department—in the early stages of your career, there are a few things you should know about each for your own decision making. You want to know about the relative standing of your group and your department if only to know if the situation serves your interests or not.

Psychologists in key disciplinary areas in a key department in a university probably have little to worry about. But if the interests of your department and university oppose your own, you would probably do well to concentrate on getting yourself into a new situation. Most people do not find their ideal jobs on the first try. The quality and attractiveness of available jobs is a matter of timing and conditions in the field upon graduation. Individually, we have little control over these. In the 1970s, job prospects were scarce, forcing painful comparisons with mentors of the 1960s who found jobs aplenty.

A bad first job, however, can be good for getting into a more attractive situation. Eventually, this is what Janet did. She quit. The special travel grant she needed was a critical reason. The conference she wanted to attend involved the major researchers in her area. A main item on the agenda was to codify important new developments, many of which were in various stages of half-finished ideas and experiments. To not attend would leave Janet out on these developments; she would have little impact in setting the field's research agenda for the next few years and would not be identified as one of its serious participants. Given this, Janet went into debt for another $1,000 and went to the conference. There she met enough people interested in her work that one of them hired her the next year. The new department was more supportive of her area in psychology, and so things ended up quite well for her. To some extent, she lucked out.

Learning the Hard Way—After the Fact

There are two ways of discovering where you stand in an organization. There is the easy way and the hard way. The hard way is after the fact. The hard way is when your political relationships get to a point of not delivering what you need. Eventually the decisions taken about you tell you very clearly that you are not what's important. It's much the same as when you make an appointment with someone who later breaks it. Excepting emergencies, a person doing this is telling you that you are not as important as something else just then.

Janet learned the hard way. The department let her know with its decisions a painful truth: It had little interest in making choices to favor her interests. How can we be so sure that Janet's misfortune signaled anything more than what the department head told her—namely, that his funds were all committed and that he wished he had known of her needs earlier? Basically one uses the same criteria used in theory testing in behavioral science. You hypothesize about what could have happened and evaluate the possibilities against what you know about what did happen.

Janet's case had many signals. One was consistency. Her failure to get what she needed happened several times in a few years. Beyond that was what the head told her. You might remember that on two occasions he mentioned that he wished he had known of her needs earlier. A kindly gesture perhaps, except that if Janet, a neophyte professor in the department, didn't know that she was supposed to ask for certain things at certain times, then it was probably because no one was telling her, neither colleagues nor the department head.

Now let's consider what the department head could have done but didn't. He could have dipped into his budget, or found funds for Janet from another source, perhaps the university administration. One must wonder why he rejected these options. If he couldn't dip into his own budget, the only reason could be that he had already committed its funds to someone he thought more of than Janet. If he didn't seek funds from the central administration, it could only mean he was not in good standing with the administration or that he did not consider Janet's request important enough to put his standing on the line. In either case Janet was a low priority.

As it turned out, things happened fairly much as hypothesized. Janet knew of the other person needing special travel funds because she spoke to him about it. He was a cognitive psychologist who entered the department with Janet. The cognitive group was the second largest area represented in the department; they supported some ten of its thirty graduate students, and had just put in for a large research program at the university. The program might or might not end up being funded from outside, but the department head was willing to risk that it would and negotiated a commitment from the central administration for initial funding. He would have been reluctant to make further requests. Janet's competitor, in the meantime, had already made his request to the department head, on the advice of one of the more seasoned faculty in his area.

Obviously, when push came to shove, Janet's case ended up on the floor, as one might predict.

Learning the Easy Way—From History

The serious mistake Janet made in her first job was not becoming aware of her situation sooner. Not to have known about the relative status of her area, the priorities of the department, the administrative details affecting the allocation of funds, all of these left her in a poor position for dealing with her department head and cultivating her interests. There's a bit of Janet in every new assistant professor. It is always surprising to discover how little people know about the places where they have committed themselves to work for 4 or 5 years at a clip. Credible psychologists who will spend hours preparing for every detail of an experiment and its analysis will spend hardly any time learning about the details of the institutions that distribute the resources needed to undertake the experiment. This is more neglect than anything else.

We describe some ways of finding out about the political situation in your department and university. It is surprisingly easy to uncover key features of most universities. Public universities are somewhat more open than private ones, and some even publish intimate details of budgetary decisions. This is a good place to look for information about how decisions have been made over the years. But pouring over budget figures can be quite tedious and in many institutions not possible.

Luckily, there are other readily available sources of information. The phone directory and course catalog are two of the most useful. When you visit an institution to interview or lecture, you might pick these up and peruse them for a few minutes to find out what's going on in the school. Look for simple indicators. Which departments are larger? What are the distributions for junior to senior faculty? Which departments have larger administrative staffs? Which departments have "institutes" or "programs" associated with them? Established institutes and programs usually indicate both special interest groups and the special sources of internal or external funding.

Members on important committees are usually listed in a directory. As we saw earlier, power structures are usually revealed by the fields represented consistently on key committees. Different institutions may name their key committees differently. In mine, they are called "promotion and tenure" and "research board" committees. But in every university, the important positions and committees are unmistakably identified by whether they handle academic budget or personnel decisions. Who is promoted and how much budget is given a department are important matters in every university community.

We can be certain that appointments to key positions reflect political structure because the matters to be dealt with cannot long ignore critical dependencies. The powerful themselves need do nothing for this to happen. Those who depend on them will eagerly include them in important matters of council. When university officials invite my department head to consume hours of boredom in a committee meeting, it is because he represents a constituency that others want to address. And when he accepts the invitation, it is because they represent constituencies he wants to address. Conspiring thus, they create the power structure.

A university's course catalog is no less a source of intelligence about its decision making. It mirrors the richness of the university's offerings, and indicates the "atmosphere" of the institution. A research-oriented department groans with lists of deadpan seminar titles. An undergraduate-oriented catalog sparkles with exciting titles on topical issues. Jim March noted about Stanford, for instance, that during turbulent and harsh times the university staved off a lot of undergraduate and faculty discontent with new course titles that appealed to the tone of the times.

The other reason for perusing course catalogs and directories is that they reveal possible sources of conflict in and between departments. A psychology department with numerous subareas has a greater potential for conflict than one with few. And one with two few subareas is likely to be one that either doesn't have sufficient resources to build a critical mass of faculty in psychology or one that has had conflict in the past and resolved it by removing or angering the weaker areas. Whatever the cause, the department will be a different place than one with a balanced set of areas represented. A department heavily weighted in one area with only a token or two in others signals a politically dominated situation. There has to be some reason for the imbalance, and a person being considered for the minority area should not jump in without finding out what it is. And if past conflicts or a lack of appreciation for the area were the source, then one might want to think carefully about whether that department was a place to be.

History as a Conversation Killer

A most important reason for appreciating the historical conditions in your institutions is because those who do understand it use it to wipe away the ignorant. You will meet such people in committee meetings. You introduce some incredibly sensible idea. You probably will have thought about it before the meeting and discussed it with colleagues. From everything you know, it is perfect. You present it. Bang! An old flatus groans with charming sympathy, "Ah yes, I like your proposal. . . . But we tried that some years back. . . . and it didn't work. Nice idea though." The room goes silent and then moves on to important matters. This happens with such frequency that it deserves thinking about how to handle it. You may have seen the same in seminars. A speaker delivers a brilliant analysis of a problem and awaits applause. Then, somebody asks, "Well, interesting idea. Didn't Sanderwall try that direction a few years back . . . and found it didn't work? The method, perhaps as Sanderwall suggested, has its flaws?" Of course, the reference would baffle top librarians.

The immediate way of avoiding such indelicacies is head-on. Ask the individual referencing the obscure past to report on what exactly was tried then and what happened. You are still at a disadvantage because you depend on the person demolishing your ideas for the recounted facts. Thus, you should go beyond asking what happened, and beyond asking this one chronicler. Find out about the circumstances. Likely as not they changed over time. And, if it's important enough, ask others in the room or suggest deferral until there is time to consider the circumstances. More prudently yet, avoid such situations by learning a bit more about the history of your institutions. A very good source of considerable information can easily be found in the newspaper archives. One can spend a productive afternoon scanning old copies of the campus paper, or employee newsletter, to find out what has been considered important and critical in the organization.

Cultivating Your Value in a University

Knowing where you stand as an assistant professor is not enough to justify your claims on resources. You also need to enhance your value to an organization by solving its problems. The problems that gain you influence have certain qualities. They must seem important and critical to your organization and your contributions to their solution should be viewed as unique. It's your uniqueness that makes you valuable, not your redundancy.

Identifying the critical problems of a department should not be too difficult. The key is to remember what creates power in the first place. Problems organize around an organization's continuing needs for resources over which it has no reliable or satisfactory control. Some of these are obvious. If you're in a research university, then graduate students are likely to create continuing problems. Funding is always a problem. But it is not the only one, and may not be the critical one. There may be too few graduate students or too many. If there are too few, developing ways of recruiting more may be useful. If there are too many, problems will arise about evaluating them and organizing research and course activities for them.

Whether yours is a research university or not, other perennial departmental needs revolve around teaching. If you are in a large department with a fairly integrated curriculum, managing the undergraduate introductory course will be a common concern for your department. Such courses usually are taught in large lectures because few faculty are motivated to teach them and few departments are willing to give up opportunities to teach other courses. Few universities, however, are fortunate enough to have a master impressario like Phil Zimbardo, whose fame as a star classroom performer spreads well beyond Stanford. Thus most departments face real and well-recognized problems about their introductory course. And the need is often continual. The people who teach it eventually tire of doing so, keeping heads on the look-out for the next generation of talented educators. Anyone who can handle this elephant for a department is likely to gain considerable gratitude from colleagues and department heads alike.

Other large lecture courses may also be a source of power for you or your disciplinary group. A large lecture course can generate thousands of instructional units for a department. They also may serve as a springboard into the department's advanced courses, a help to faculty in other areas as well as your own. Honors programs are yet another place to make teaching contributions. They take time, but, depending on how well they are handled, can also aid a department's recruiting needs by feeding its doctoral program.

The point is that there are many contributions one can make that are strategically important for a department. What they can be in your institution is something you should be creative about. Few departments are without a long list of nagging problems they know they should be working on but never quite get around to doing. Most of these involve tasks requiring only creative thought. Or they demand a practical energy or administrative skill. Sometimes they are just things that get put aside from year to year. A good candidate in most departments is doctoral students recruiting. During good years, applicants flood in and there is no problem. In lean years, the lack of qualified prospects occasions panic. But comes the fall term, the crisis is over and everyone forgets about it until the next spring. Depending on the circumstances in your department, this is the kind of problem that might earn both visibility and respect from colleagues. Usually they don't take as much real time to solve as people think, mostly attention. Perhaps a brochure might be an answer. Perhaps a simple encouraging letter to honor students.

Some cautions about selecting how you will contribute are also in order. Certainly you want to avoid activities that take you away from your main academic purpose. However encouraging departments may appear at the prospect of a thorn being removed, they never forgive young scholars who let their research slide. Sometimes they'll put you in a double bind. It's not because they're pernicious. It usually follows an innocent desire to encourage your initiative and an erroneous assumption that you wouldn't be foolish enough to take on extra work if you didn't have the rest of your life in perfect order.

Assuming you do have your life in order, you should try to do things that suit your skills, interfere little with other goals, and gain you visibility. As a corollary, be sure the credit goes to you when it is done. Don't be rude in taking credit, but don't be rash in giving it away. One department head told us that it is grating to hear, "If I teach a service course, I want a higher salary," but not "I'll be glad to teach the course, though it means I'll spend a good part of the summer preparing. Is there a possibility for summer salary, or could it somehow be built into my regular salary?"

One activity that meets all the criteria as a suitable role for new faculty members is running a colloquium or proseminar series. This can be a benefit in several ways. It is often prominent within and outside a department, since most faculty and students in active departments attend, and if they haven't been lately you can usually embarrass them to do so at least once. Running a lecture series is also minimally distracting to a research program. It actually takes little time to do, the biggest problems being scheduling and telephoning prospective speakers and informing your colleagues of the events. Moreover, it puts you in contact with members in your field and is a pleasant way to introduce yourself to them. Even if people turn you down, most are flattered to have been asked. Finally, coordinating the visits of speakers grants you a perfectly legitimate reason to meet your own faculty and gives you a chance to learn about them and they about you.

Cultivating Your Value Outside

Although you can do many things for your department directly, your main value will come from what you accomplish outside it. Recall that academic units created their power by the resources they brought to the university. This is as true at the departmental level. Valued faculty in psychology departments are also likely to be valued in their fields. Their roles in their fields lend many things to a department, not least of which is reassurance of its faculty's quality. Well-known or well-connected faculty bring in contacts and information that may aid decisions of either individuals or the department as a whole. Mostly, they bring in prestige as a direct or indirect result of their research and the role they play in their subarea of psychology.

When your research program is just starting out, it is difficult to contribute great amounts of prestige. But it is not too soon to begin developing the relationships upon which reputations rely. Reputations are social not scientific phenomena. They follow when people believe that what you do is good. To gain a reputation, several things have to happen. You have to create something and, then, others have to hear about it, have to judge it to be worthwhile and have to tell still others that they think so. Note your role is minor compared to the roles of others. That puts you in a very disadvantaged position, but you are not powerless. You just need to be very clear about the role others play and work from there. Next we discuss some facets of this process—networks and your contributions to them.

Power in Scientific and Resource Networks

If you read the psychological pap that follows the baby boom generation around, you surely must know by now that you should be "networking." If you are shy as I am, however, you probably feel more than slightly intimidated at the prospect that you must, in addition to becoming a great scholar, spend hours on the telephone passing privy trade news and tips about ensuing moves and prospects about the fine and the famous in your field. You might also shudder with regret as you stand, alongside me, in your corner of the convention floor during the cocktail hour watching your engagingly witty colleagues poised with note pads jotting their addresses for the eager inviting them to upcoming colloquia or wanting them on a mailing list.

Well, rest assured. You already belong to many networks, and others that you might need you can easily create. A network is just that—a network. If it is a well-connected network, then, theoretically, you can access it at any point and retrieve from it all the other points. The points represent people. And the people represent bundles of resources—resources like information, access to positions and opportunities, administrative skill, methodological skill, creative and analytic skill, and skill in rendering evaluative judgment. From these there emerge, from time to time, coalitions that organize symposia, collaborators that create new research programs, and climates of opinion that pass on reputations and prestige. To become a point in a network requires only that you have resources to contribute and that you know at least one other point in the network. If the network is efficient and the resources you have to contribute are valuable, people will be in contact with you. You will not even have to jot your address down for them, as they will get it from those who already know you. In an efficient network, if one member needed someone to write a review chapter and you were the most appropriate person to conduct the review, you would be the one asked to write it.

Unfortunately, networks are not efficient. Mostly this is because the resource contributions of each member are not unique. Many needs can be satisfied by several members. Yet your value to the network is a function of the uniqueness and importance of your own resources. Another reason that networks are not efficient, however, is because they contain shysters and brokers. Shysters misrepresent the resources they possess and, thereby, diminish the uniqueness of your potential contributions. They wittingly engage book editors and end up writing your book chapter. Brokers try to horde access points to the network; they get to know as many members as they can, hoping to force everyone to go through them for resources. This obviously makes them very important to the extent they are successful. They are the ones that we shy people notice writing down their own telephone numbers rather than the name of the person who could write the chapter needed by a prospecting editor. The reason is because they want to ring up the chapter writer themselves, pass on the good news, and get full credit for making the contact. Sensible people, but once they connect two members, their role as a broker ends since the parties now know one another. To retain their positions, then, brokers constantly introduce new people into the network. The network expands and your uniqueness in it diminishes.

Clearly we shy people have good reason to dislike glib colleagues. They leave us only one recourse: To restrict our networks to those where we are most valued. The trick to participating successfully in a network is to have it as small and as relevant to your interests as possible. For professional purposes, one needs only two kinds of networks—colleagues who share your scientific interests and the elite in a discipline who allocate its opportunities and prestige. The first defines the second so we'll begin there.

Creating Your Own Network

Whether you are shy or not, you begin developing a network by identifying the individuals relevant to you. You may already have them in mind. They are the people whose work most closely relates to your own. They should be on both sides of your intellectual fence—those whose theories agree with and oppose yours. The list should be no more than 10 to 20 individuals. Of those, note the five persons most critical to the development of your research area in the next years. The number five is arbitrary except in the direction of its magnitude. If you have selected correctly, some of them would also have selected you for their lists and, given the chance, review and cite your work. Although the ones you've chosen may not yet know your work, they would be the ones most motivated to do so in the future. On your second list will be individuals who are somewhat interested in your work, or whose work you may be interested in getting into in the future. Ignore it for now.

The five people you've identified are the ones you respect and want to get to know, if you do not already. Obviously, you want them to appreciate you. A reliable fact from social psychology is that if you like them, behave decently towards them and show respect for their work, they will have no difficulty liking you. You can let them know with a short note saying so. Very short, "Read your paper (title) and wonder if you have done any additional work that you would be willing to send me. Thank you." Nothing else, except your address for mailing the paper. Do this a few times at respectable intervals and you will have communicated your respect, interest, and suitability as an appropriate colleague. If an individual doesn't respond by sending anything, drop the person from your list and add another from your reserve list. If one responds by sending work long available in the literature, write back acknowledging your familiarity and asking about more recent developments. If none come, replace the person with another from your list.

Read the material sent you and comment on it if asked. Depending on the extent of the interest expressed and your own ease in these matters, send them a piece of your own work when you have something that you think is seriously relevant to theirs. In addition, mention the works you receive to others on your list for whom it is relevant. Continue this until you feel comfortable in knowing these colleagues. By this time, you will have a good feel for their interest in you. Let them know about upcoming events of common scientific interest and ask about their attendance. Plan to meet at general conventions or conferences. Ask for advice on technical or theoretical issues as you plan your own work. Ask for advice on grant proposals. If you have the resources, or control your department's colloquium series, invite one or another to give a talk at your university. If you have the resources, visit them. If something useful is generated on these occasions, pass it on to the others who were absent.

Continuing in this vein for a year or so, you will have organized a network most directly relevant to your interests. As your experience in doing this expands, add more names to the list. Some will come from your new colleagues. Others will come from your first list. However, only add them if they are relevant. Drop any that become disinterested in your work or that you misidentified initially. In a year or so, the remaining, their colleagues, and you collectively constitute the network of your area in psychology. There is likely to be some of the elite among them. Some will be the intellectual ancestors of your specialty. Or they may be the grant review panel members that fund your area. Or they may be potential reviewers of your papers. You probably have no need to wonder if you should approach them at meetings, because they already know you, having been introduced to you either through your correspondence or through your colleagues'. Your colleagues, by following your example, will have extended to you the same courtesies you showed them. The most important result of this investment, however, is that you and this group over time will have constructed a social consensus about the work you are all doing.

Crunched together in a description as we have done here, this may seem like a lot of work. Over time, however, it is very little work. And the little time it takes to develop your relationships with colleagues will pay off in terms of your interests, if you selected only those with your interests in the first place.

POLITICS AND THE POLITIC IN USING YOUR POWER

With all this attention to power in academia, you might wonder if you should get involved in all kinds of political activity in your department and the other institutions of psychology that affect you. By politics we mean any effort you take to influence decisions towards your preferences.

Actually, we have only one piece of advice, and it follows everything we have said. Get involved in the politics of your institutions as little as possible and never unless your interests are seriously at stake. It takes more time than it is worth to you, because every effort you make fighting battles that are not in your interests is taking time from your interests. Most decisions are in somebody's interest; those for whom serious issues are at stake will put more energy into it than you, know more about it, and quite likely have more legitimate claims, all of which put them in a position to get their way over yours. You may only end up becoming what is known technically by administrators, and other regulators of the public weal, as a PITA—a pain in the ass. Your effectiveness plunges accordingly.

Our view is more structural. If you have to argue your case, you've lost too much of it already. Better advice is to manage your desires, accept the dependencies you can rely on, and create the social networks where the things you do are valued.

ACKNOWLEDGMENTS

Thanks to many friends and two stern and clever editors, this chapter was possible.

II HANDLING CRITICAL ELEMENTS OF AN ASSISTANT PROFESSORSHIP

4

TIPS ON TEACHING

W. J. McKeachie
University of Michigan

Most faculty members report that they like teaching. Surveys of college and university faculty find that faculty members would like to have more time for teaching. Yet we have all encountered professors who seemed dull, uninterested in their courses, and hostile toward students.

What accounts for the gap between teaching at its best and poor teaching? Why do some teachers never develop a love of teaching?

I would argue that the first few months and years of teaching are all-important. Experiences during this period can blight a promising teaching career or can start one on a path of continued growth and development.

Most of us go into our first classes as teachers with a good deal of fear and trembling. We don't want to appear to be fools; so we have prepared well, but we dread the embarrassment of not being able to answer students' questions. We want to be liked and respected by our students; yet we know that we have to achieve liking and respect in a new role which carries expectations, such as evaluation, that make our relationship with students edgy and uneasy. We want to get through the first class with eclat but we don't know how much material we can cover in a class period.

Thus the first days and weeks and months of teaching are fraught with anxiety. In most cases the anxiety passes as one finds that students do respond positively, that one does have some expertise in the subject, and that class periods can be exciting. But for some teachers the first days are not happy experiences. Classes get off on the wrong foot. Sullen hostility sets in. The teacher asserts authority and the students resist. The teacher knows that things are not going well but doesn't know what to do about it.

One likely response is retreat—retreat to reading lectures with as little eye contact with students as possible—retreat to threats of low grades as a motivating device—retreat to research and other aspects of the professorial role.

What makes the difference in these first few days? Frequently a few simple skills.

The new teacher who has techniques for breaking the ice, for encouraging class participation, for getting the course organized is more likely to get off to a good start. Once one finds that teaching can be fun, one is likely to enjoy devoting time to it, and if one devotes that time, one will develop into a competent teacher. Anyone bright enough to complete a graduate degree is bright enough to learn the skills and concepts needed for effective teaching.

What can I do to help you get off to a good start? Perhaps simply pass on ideas that have been helpful to me. Some of them won't fit your course or your style, but some may stimulate you to develop your own adaptation in a way that will make teaching more fun.

Coming into a New Institution

Most of us teach as we have been taught. If most of our courses in college have been lectures, we lecture. If we come from a department that used a case study approach, we use the case method. If our own undergraduate courses used films, we plan to use films.

But the culture, the teaching norms, differ from college to college. You risk embarrassment and frustration if you start out on the assumption that your new place of employment expects the same sort of teaching behavior as that characterizing your undergraduate and graduate institutions.

What can you do? Well, you could visit classes. That in itself is such rare behavior that it is likely to be deviant. Nonetheless you'll find that most of your new colleagues are flattered by your request to learn by observing them.

Even if class visitation isn't possible, it will still pay to talk to your new colleagues. Ask! What do you do in teaching here? What teaching methods are prevalent? How are students graded? What about textbooks, syllabi, teaching aids, term papers, library references, laboratories, or fieldwork? How much work outside of class can you expect students to do? What office hours are you expected to keep?

Look at syllabi. Find out as much as possible about how your courses have been taught in the past and what changes the department would like to see. Get copies of the syllabus in your course and those related to it. Check out the library and the film catalog. And when students tell you, "Other professors do this or that," don't automatically accept their statements as accurate representations of the culture.

Most colleges and universities tolerate great variability in faculty behavior, but when you deviate, it is better to know that you are de and that you are doing it for a good reason rather than blundering because you hadn't realized that there was a way different from that you have experienced.

Be particularly alert to find grading norms. Nothing is more sacred to college faculties than grading standards. The easy grader must perforce be a poor scholar. And even sex and alcohol are less serious matters to students than grades so that the faculty member who is an unusually hard grader must be prepared for student grievances.

In short, if you're to get a good start in teaching, "you've got to know the territory."

Broadening Your Perspective

Your new colleagues should be your best informed and most supportive sources of help. But approaching colleagues with questions about teaching involves some risk. They can be helpful, but they also are evaluators. Sometime not too distant they may be asked to vote on your promotion. Your situation is much like that of the students in your class who want to understand but are afraid that revealing their ignorance will result in a lower grade. Don't be put off. Faculty members like to be appealed to for advice. Most have few opportunities to talk about teaching. Your question will be more often welcomed as a chance to share experience than as an interruption. In addition to colleagues, there are other sources of help. My book, *Teaching Tips,* 7th edition, D. C. Heath, has been used by beginning faculty members for over 30 years. Within the last few years a number of excellent books on college teaching have appeared. Here are a few that I like:

Erickson, S. C. Jossey-Bass, In press.
Furhman, B. & Grasha, A. *A Practical Handbook for College Teachers,* Little Brown, 1983.
Lohman, F. *Mastering the Techniques of Teaching.* Jossey-Bass, 1984.
Dressel P. & Marcus, D. *On Teaching and Learning in College*. Jossey-Bass, 1982.

If you're teaching an introductory course, ask Scott Foresman to send you a desk copy of Zimbardo's *Psychology and Life* with the Instructor's Manual. The Instructor's Manual lays out the stages in course planning from three months before to the first day of class.

So you've planned your course; you have a syllabus. Give it to one of your new colleagues to look over. Be prepared to revise it, not only on the basis of colleague reactions but later as you see how it works out in practice. At some point it has to be duplicated for the students but this should not mean that it is immutable. Frequent, unpremeditated changes make the students restless, but the syllabus should provide a framework, not a straitjacket.

One point, however, about deviations from the syllabus—or even more important from the college norms. Explain to the students what the goal is of the change. Try to make clear what they will need to do and what they will get out of it.

Now You Have a Syllabus, What Next?

Preparation and planning are not done when you've firmed up the syllabus. Now look back over the syllabus to see what resources are required. Presumably your check with a colleague has turned up any gross problems—such as assuming an unlimited budget for films. But visit the classroom you've been assigned. Will the seating be conducive to discussion? Can it be darkened for films? If the room is unsuitable, ask for another. Don't assume that assignments are unchangeable. You probably can't change the time schedule the first time you are assigned it, since a certain time may already be in print with student schedules built around it. But with a term's head start you may be able to shift time of day, length of class period, and so forth. What are the library policies relevant to putting on reserve any books you may want to reserve? Can you assume unlimited xeroxing of exams and course materials to give to students? What do you do if you want to show a film? Go on a field trip?

Teaching Style

A less concrete aspect of course preparation is to think about the styles and methods of teaching that are best suited to the course goals, type of students, classroom, and your own skills and personality. The lecture is not always the best method for all undergraduate classes—not even for large introductory classes. You can build large-group discussion methods, pairs, buzz groups, or other methods into large courses. And even within the lecture method there are great opportunities for stylistic variations. If you have a sense of humor, let it out; if you have an earnest interest in your subject and teaching, let the students see it.

Don't feel you have to tell jokes if you're not a natural comedian, but don't get settled into a rut of a limited style and method. Teaching is a developmental activity, and you can develop and learn new skills that broaden your repertoire.

LECTURING

The lecture[1] is probably the oldest teaching method and still the method most widely used in North American colleges and universities. Through the ages a great deal of practical wisdom about techniques of lecturing has accumulated. Effective lecturers combine the talents of scholar, writer, producer, comedian, showman, and teacher in ways that contribute to student learning. Nevertheless, it is also true that few college professors combine these talents in optimal ways and that even the best lecturers are not always in top form.

One way of improving lectures is to think about how students process lectures. What are students trying to do during a lecture?

As one looks at students at a lecture and observes their behavior, the most impressive thing one notices is the passive role students have in most classrooms. Some students are having difficulty in staying awake; others are attempting to pass the time as easily as possible by reading other materials, counting lecturer mannerisms, or simply doodling and listening in a relatively effortless manner. Many students are taking notes. In most cases, when queried about their listening or note-taking habits, they report that they are primarily concerned about getting the gist of the lecture in order to be prepared for an examination. To do this they try to extract significant features from the lecture, to distill some of its meaning.

Hartley and Davies (1978) reviewed the research on note-taking and student information-processing during lectures. They report that students believe that there are two purposes for taking notes: one is that the process of taking notes will in itself help later recall; the other is that the notes provide external storage of concepts which may be reviewed when needed. The research results indicate some support for both beliefs, but note-taking has costs as well as benefits. Student strategies of note-taking differ. Some students take copious notes; others take none. We know that student information processing capacity is limited; that is, people can take in, understand, and store only so much information in any brief period of time. Information will be processed more effectively if the student is actively engaged in processing the information rather than passively soaking it up. Students' ability to process information depends upon the degree to which the information can be integrated or "chunked." No one has great ability at handling large numbers of unrelated items in active memory. Thus when students are in an area in which there are many new concepts or when the instructor is using language that is not entirely familiar to the students, students may be processing the lecture word by word or phrase by phrase and lose the sense of a sentence or of a paragraph before the end of the thought is reached. This means that lecturers need to be aware of instances in which new words or concepts are being introduced and to build in greater redundancy as well as pauses during which students can catch up and get appropriate notes.

Brighter students benefit more from taking notes than less able students, and we believe that this is because the less able students are not able, while they write their notes, to keep what they hear in their memories, so that their note-taking essentially blocks them from processing parts of the lecture. But this is not simply a matter of intelligence; rather a student's ability to maintain materials in memory while taking notes and even to process and think about relationships between one idea and other ideas depends upon the knowledge or cognitive structures the student has available for organizing and relating the material. Thus the background of the student in the area is probably more important than the students' level of intelligence.

Attention

One of the factors determining students' information-processing is their ability to attend to the lecture. We know that individuals have a limited capacity for attending to the varied features of their environment. The individual's total capacity for attention may vary with the degree of activation or motivation. At any one time, part of the capacity is devoted to the task at hand (in this case listening to the lecturer), part is monitoring other aspects of the classroom, and part of the attention capacity may be available for other uses—in other words, it is simply spare capacity.

In determining how to allocate attention, students use various strategies. Any lecturer knows that one way of getting attention is to precede the statement by the phrase, "This will be on the test." In addition, students listen for particular words or phrases that indicate to them that something is worth noting and remembering. Statements that enumerate or list points are likely to be on tests and thus are likely to be attended to.

Changes in the environment recruit attention. The ability of changes to capture attention can work to the advantage of the lecturer. Variation in pitch, intensity, and pace of the lecture, and visual cues such as gestures, facial expression, movement to the blackboard, the use of demonstrations or audio-visual aids—all of these recruit and maintain attention to the lecture.

Hartley and Davies' review of research notes that, typically, attention increases from the beginning of the lecture to ten minutes into the lecture and decreases after that point. One evidence of this was that after the lecture students recalled 70% of the material covered in the first 10 minutes, and only 20% of the material covered in the last 10 minutes.

Auditory attention is directed to some extent by visual attention. As the eyes move, auditory attention tends to shift as well. Distracting movements in the classroom are likely to cause students to fail to recall what the lecturer has said. On the positive side, there is some evidence that students' comprehension is greater when the students can see the speaker's face and lips. Thus attempts of colleges and universities to conserve energy by reducing the lighting level may also reduce the students' abilities to maintain attention and learn from the lecture.

One of the characteristics of a passive lecture situation in which a lecturer is using few devices to get students to think actively about the content of the lecture is that attention tends to drift. Probably all of us have had the experience of listening to a speaker and finding with a start that we have not heard the speaker for some time because our attention has drifted on to thoughts that are tangential to the lecturer's theme. Bloom's (1953) studies of students' thinking during lectures and discussions indicated that more of students' thoughts were relevant to the content during lectures than during discussions, but that there was less active thinking in lectures than in discussions.

I previously indicated that at most times when students are not highly motivated there is spare capacity of attention available. This spare capacity is very likely to be used for daydreaming or other tasks which may become more engrossing than listening to the lecture.

Another factor determining the amount of capacity devoted to monitoring the lecture is anxiety. There is a good deal of evidence that students who are high in anxiety about tests are likely during tests to fail to pay attention to the test because they are distracted by thought of failure (Wine, 1971). It seems likely that such anxiety about achievement may also distract a student listening to a lecture. In fact some of the very cues used by the lecturer to attract attention, such as "this will be on the test," may also cue anxious thoughts about the likelihood of failing the test, about the consequences of failing in college and the resulting disappointment of family. Thus, while heavy emphasis upon tests and grades may cause some students to increase the amount of attention devoted to the lecture, it may also negatively affect others to the degree that their thoughts turn to the consequences of success or failure.

ORGANIZATION OF LECTURES

In thinking about lecture organization, most teachers think first about the structure of the subject matter, then try to organize the content in some logical fashion, such as building from specifics to generalizations or deriving specific implications from general principles. There is a danger in considering your lecture organization solely in terms of communication of information. As you think about preparing lectures keep in mind that stimulating motivation is probably even more important than information transmission. Your task is to intrigue student interest and stimulate *their* thinking, not simply to give them the results of your thinking.

Some common organizing principles used by lecturers are cause to effect; time sequence (for example, stories); phenomena to theory to evidence; problem to solution; pro versus con to resolution; familiar to unfamiliar; and concept to application.

Leith (1977) has suggested that different subjects are basically different in the ways in which progress is made in the field. Some subjects are organized in a linear or hierarchical fashion in which one concept builds upon a preceding one. In such subjects one must follow a particular sequence of ideas in order to reach a sophisticated level. Other subject matters are organized more nearly in the manner of a spiral or helix in which the path from one level to the next is not linear but rather depends on accumulating a number of related ideas before the next level can be achieved; and any of the related ideas at one level need not precede other ideas at that level. Still other subject matters are organized in the fashion of networks in which one may start at different points of the network and go in various directions. One may build up a network equally well by starting at any one of a number of places and proceeding through a variety of sequences to arrive at comprehension of the subject matter.

The logical structure of one's subject should be one factor determining the lecture organization, but probably equally as important as the structure of the subject matter is the cognitive structure in the students' minds. If we are to teach our students effectively, we need to bridge the gap between the structure in the subject matter and structures in the students' minds. The learner's mind is not a *tabula rasa;* the teacher is not making impressions on a blank slate. Rather our task in teaching is to recognize existing student cognitive structures or to add new dimensions or new features to existing structures. Thus the organization of the lecture needs to take account of the students' existing knowledge, expectations, and interests as well as the structure of the subject matter.

The Introduction

One suggestion for organization is that the *introduction* of the lecture should point to a gap in the student's existing cognitive structure or should challenge or raise a question about something in the student's existing method of organizing material in order to arouse curiosity

(Berlyne, 1954). There is a good deal of research on the role of prequestions in directing attention to features of written texts. Prequestions in the introduction of a lecture may help students to discriminate between more or less important features of lectures. For example, before a lecture on cognitive changes in aging, I ask, "Do you get more or less intelligent as you get older?" "What would be a fair test of intelligence for older people?" Such questions may also help to create expectations which will enable the students to allocate their information-processing capacity more effectively. If students know what they are expected to learn from a lecture, they learn more (Royer, 1977).

Body of the Lecture

In organizing the *body* of the lecture, the most common error is probably that of trying to include too much. As we have stressed throughout this chapter, students' information-processing capacities are limited, and a lecturer who is expert in the field is likely to overestimate the students' ability to grasp large blocks of material and to see relationships. Relationships that seem obvious to an expert in the field are not obvious to students, and thus lecturers very often overload the students' capacity so that they become less able to understand than if fewer points had been presented. David Katz (1950), a pioneer Gestalt psychologist, called this phenomenon "mental dazzle." Just as too much light causes our eyes to be dazzled so that we cannot see anything, so too, too many new ideas can overload processing capacity so that we cannot understand anything.

It seems likely that students will differ in their ability to benefit from particular kinds of sequences. As Mayer and Greeno (1972) have shown, some students do better when they are given a sequence of generalizations first and specific drill and practice sequences second, whereas other students do better when the specifics lead to generalizations.

Whatever the structure one uses, it is clear from research that highlighting the structure and giving students cues to the nature of organization that one is using is helpful to many students, particularly those who are lower in intelligence or more anxious (Snow & Peterson, 1980). Davis's studies of outstanding lecturers (1976) indicated that professors known as outstanding lecturers did two things: they used a simple plan and many examples.

Periodic Summaries Within the Lecture

From our knowledge of students' note-taking behavior and from our theory of information processing, it seems likely that students would be better able to learn from lectures if there were periodic summaries of preceding material. These give students a chance to catch up on material covered when they were not tuned in and also give them a check upon possible misperceptions based upon inadequate or misleading expectations. Moreover, such summaries can help make clear to students transitions from one theme to another so that they are aided in organizing the material not only in their notes but in their minds.

Probably one of the greatest barriers to effective lecturing is the feeling that one must cover the material at all costs. Although it may seem irrational to cover material when students are not learning from it, one should not underestimate the compulsion one feels to get through one's lecture notes. A remedy for this compulsion is to put into the lecture notes reminders to oneself to check the students' understanding—both by looking for nonverbal cues of bewilderment or lack of attention and by raising specific questions that will test the students' understanding. I also put in the margins reminders to myself to put key words or topic headings on the blackboard. This not only provides movement and a visual stimulus to capture student attention, but also helps students get a better sense of your organization. Hartley found that providing complete notes encouraged student passivity, but with no cues to organization some students get lost.

The Conclusion

In the conclusion of the lecture, one has the opportunity to make up for lapses in the body of the lecture. Encouraging students to formulate questions or asking questions oneself can facilitate understanding and memory. By making the oral headings visible once again, by recapitulating major points, by proposing unanswered questions to be treated in the reading assignments or the future lectures, and by creating an anticipation of the future, the lecturer can help students learn. Having suggested all this, I must admit that my own greatest problem as a lecturer is that I never seem to be ready for the conclusion until it is already time to dismiss the class.

THE SEMINAR

One of the most common formats for advanced undergraduate and graduate courses is the seminar. Unfortunately too many faculty members take the seminar as a chance to relax and let the students do the work. Both relaxation and student work are laudable aspects of good seminars, but seminars frequently fail because of a lack of energy and planning. Ideally seminars involve opportunities for all the students as well as the teacher to contribute knowledge and ideas to the topics of the seminar. For this to occur all participants need some common basis of information. The student presenting should not simply read a prepared paper, but rather should attempt to develop conclusions or issues that will stimulate active involvement of all members of the seminar. I typically handle the first few topics myself, while getting students (or teams of students) signed up promptly to be responsible for topics after the first two or three weeks. Each team is not only responsible for leading discussion on "their day" but also for providing a paper of suggested reading for the other students to study in advance of the discussion. I've found that it pays to meet with each team both to assist them in getting to sources and to consider how to elicit and facilitate effective discussion. Done well the seminar can be a fine learning experience both for the students and for you.

LEADING DISCUSSIONS

Discussion methods are among the most valuable tool in the teacher's repertoire. Often teachers in large classes feel that they must lecture because discussion is impossible. In fact discussion techniques can be used in classes of all sizes. This is not to say that small classes are not desirable—they *are* generally more effective, but large classes should not be allowed to inhibit the teacher's ability to stimulate student thinking and participation.

When Do We Use Discussion?

Not when we want to communicate lots of information to motivated students with a good background. But that negative answer implies part of the positive answer to our question. Discussions can be useful for developing motivation and for assessing student readiness for learning. It is also useful when we want to:

1. Help students learn to think in terms of the subject matter by giving them practice in thinking.
2. Help students learn to evaluate the logic of, and evidence for, their own and others' positions.
3. Give students opportunities to formulate applications of principles.
4. Help students become aware of and formulate problems using information to be gained from readings or lectures.
5. Use the experience or knowledge of members of the group.
6. Gain acceptance for information or theories counter to folklore or to previous beliefs of students.

7. Develop motivation for further learning.
8. Get prompt feedback on how well objectives are being attained.

In most classes we talk too much, and the students are too passive. In large classes break up your lectures with some large-group discussion techniques. In classes of 35 or fewer students where there is a decent text you'll be more effective if discussion predominates.

DISCUSSION METHODS

The type of discussion method used will determine the extent to which particular roles are dominant. Discussion methods range from recitation, in which the instructor aks specific questions in an oral quiz, to nondirective methods, in which the instructor says very little and students determine the topic and content of discussion. Generally speaking the freer discussion methods result in more impact upon attitudes and motivation and greater improvement in thinking.

Developmental Discussion

The term *developmental discussion* was coined by Professor Norman R. F. Maier (1952) to describe a problem-solving discussion technique in which the teacher breaks problems into parts so that all group members are working on the same part of the problem at the same time. One of the reasons discussion often seems ineffective and disorganized is that different members of the group are working on different aspects of the problem and are thus often frustrated by what they perceive as irrelevant comments by other students. In developmental discussion the teacher tries to keep the students aware of the step of discussion that is the current focus. Typical steps might be (a) formulating the problem; (b) suggesting hypotheses; (c) getting relevant data, and (d) evaluating alternative solutions.

Typically, an early step in developmental discussion is to get information relevant to the problem for discussion. Such information can be supplied by a lecture, reading, or group members. In developmental discussion teachers should feel free to give information or raise questions. They do not ask questions to which they already know the answers.

Like other discussion methods, developmental discussion implies active participation of group members. In developmental discussion, participation is directed to a definite goal. However, this does not imply a type of discussion leadership in which the leader manipulates the group to follow the steps and reach a predetermined goal. Rather, the leader helps the group progress by dividing the problem into parts that can be solved in steps. In short, developmental discussion is not nondirective, but neither is it autocratic.

Breaking a Problem into Subproblems

One of Maier's important contributions to effective group problem solving as well as to teaching by developmental discussion is to point out that groups are likely to be more effective if they tackle one aspect of a problem at a time rather than skipping from formulation of the problem, to solutions, to evidence, to "what-have-you," as different members of the group toss in their own ideas. In developmental discussion the group tackles one thing at a time. You might start a developmental discussion by a question such as, *Is cramming effective?* One of the first tasks is likely to be a *clarification of the problem.* Often groups are ineffective because different participants have different ideas of what the problem is, and group members may feel frustrated at the end of the discussion because "the group never got to the real problem."

In our discussion of cramming, we might first determine what we mean by cramming and what criteria we will accept for effectiveness—passing an exam? long-term retention? later use in problem solving?

A second task is likely to be, *What do we know?* or, *What data are relevant?*

A third task may be, *What are the characteristics of an acceptable solution?*—for example, *What is needed?*

A fourth step could be, *What are possible solutions?* and a fifth step may be to evaluate these solutions against the criteria for a solution determined in the previous step.

Under what conditions is cramming effective? For what goals?

The developmental discussion technique can be used even in large groups, since there are a limited number of points to be made at each step regardless of the number of participants. Maier and Maier (1957) have shown that developmental discussion techniques improve the quality of decisions as compared with freer, more nondirective discussion methods.

Skills in Leading Discussion

In a developmental discussion the teacher attempts to guide a discussion along a certain line, but not to push it beyond the group's interest and acceptance. Obviously this requires skill in initiating discussion, getting student participation, appraising group progress, asking questions, and overcoming resistance.

Starting Discussion

After a class has been meeting and discussing problems successfully, there is little problem in initiating discussion, for it will develop almost spontaneously from problems encountered in outside reading or experiences or from continuation of discussion of unresolved problems from the previous meeting. But during the first meetings of new groups, the instructor may need to assume the initiative in beginning the discussion.

Starting with a Common Experience

One of the best ways of starting a discussion is to provide a concrete, common experience through presentation of a demonstration, film, or role playing. Following such a presentation it's easy to ask, "Why did———?"

Such an opening has a number of advantages. Since everyone in the group has a common experience, everyone knows something about the topic under discussion. In addition, by focusing the discussion on the demonstration, the instructor takes some of the pressure off anxious or threatened students who are afraid to reveal their own opinions or feelings.

However, you will not always be able to find the demonstration you need to introduce each discussion; thus you may be forced to turn to other techniques of initiating discussion. One such technique is Problem Posting.

Problem Posting

The technique of posting problems[2] is not only a useful icebreaker, but one of value whenever it is useful to stimulate interest and assist students in communicating their problems to one another. This may be the case not only at the beginning of the course, but also after a lecture or other classroom method has aroused anxiety or defensiveness. The technique may also be useful to you when you wish to avoid answering questions immediately yourself. This might be because you don't wish to be placed on the defensive, because you wish to lay more groundwork, or because you don't wish to reinforce or to engage in a colloquy with a particular questioner whose concerns are not likely to contribute toward achievement of the goals of the class as a whole.

Do these potentialities intrigue you? All the discussion leader need do is to say something like, "Let's see if we can get all the questions out so that we can see what they are and how to handle them."

If it is the first class meeting, you might say, "Let's see what problems you'd like to have us tackle during the course. What sorts of concerns do you think that we might deal with?"

The instructor's task then becomes that of undestanding and recording briefly on the blackboard the problems contributed by the group. This means that you must be ready to accept all contributions whether or not you yourself feel they are important. To test your understanding of the problem it is useful to restate the problem in different words, although this technique may lead participants to feel that you are critical of the way they stated the problem. Tell the group in the beginning that you will be restating questions to test your own understanding, not because you state the problems better than anyone else. Restatement may also be useful in removing emotional loading or in bringing out implicit feelings. When you feel that a question is ambiguous or too general, it is helpful to ask for an illustration or to ask other group members to help you understand.

As contributions begin to slow down, it is often helpful to suggest stopping after a few more. But, if possible, the posting should not be ended before there has been a good pause, since some of the most deeply felt problems will not come out until the student has seen that the teacher is really accepting and noncritical of the problems raised. This is a point where sensitivity is particularly important, for one can often see the visible signs of conflict about whether or not to raise an emotion-laden problem. If such a problem does come out and elicits a new batch of problems, forget about the suggested ending and get the problems out.

It is important in problem posting to maintain an accepting, nonevaluative atmosphere. Thus, if other members of the group argue that someone's contribution is not really a problem or that the real problem is different from that stated, the leader needs to make it clear that even though not everyone agrees about a given problem, anything that is a problem for any member of the group is entitled to be listed. Disagreement should be used to get additional problems out rather than to persuade a group member to withdraw his or her contribution.

Inevitably some discussion will come out about solutions. Although this should not be abruptly censored, if it becomes involved or lengthy the teacher may point out that the task of dealing with the problems comes later.

By the end of the problem posting the class normally has become better acquainted, has become used to active participation, has taken the first step toward developing an attitude of attempting to understand rather than compete with one another, has reduced the attitude that everything must come from the teacher, has learned that the teacher can listen as well as talk and is not going to reject ideas different from his or her own, and, I hope, has begun to feel some responsibility for solving its own problems rather than waiting for them to be answered by the instructor.

Starting Discussion With a Question

There are times when it is appropriate to check student background knowledge with a series of brief factual questions, but more frequently you want to stimulate problem solving. One common error in question-phrasing for this purpose is to ask a question in a form conveying to students the message, "I know something you don't know and you'll look stupid if you don't guess right." Rather than dealing with factual questions, discussions need to be formulated so as to get at relationships, applications, or analyses of facts and materials. Solomon, Rosenberg, and Bezdek (1964) found that teachers who used interpretation questions were effective as measured by gains in student comprehension. A question of the type, "How does the idea that ——— apply to ——— ?" is much more likely to stimulate discussion than the question, "What is the definition of ——— ?" The question may arise from a case; it may be a hypothetical problem. It may be a problem whose solution the instructor knows; it may be a problem that the instructor has not solved him- or herself. In any case it should be a problem that is meaningful to the students and, for the sake of morale, it should be a problem the students can make some progress on. And even if the teacher knows an answer or has a preferred solution, the students should have a chance to come up with new solutions. The teacher's job usually is not to sell students on a particular solution, but rather to teach them how to solve problems themselves. As Maier has shown in his studies of group leadership, one barrier to problem solving is presenting an issue in such a way that participants take sides arguing the apparent solution rather than attempting to solve the problem by considering data and devising alternative solutions. Maier suggests the following principles for group problem solving:

1. Success in problem solving requires that effort be directed toward overcoming surmountable obstacles.
2. Available facts should be used even when they are inadequate.
3. The starting point of the problem is richest in solution possibilities.
4. Problem-mindedness should be increased whereas solution-mindedness should be delayed.
5. Disagreement can lead either to hard feelings or to innovation depending on the discussion leadership.
6. The "idea-getting" process should be separated from the "idea-evaluation" process because the latter inhibits the former.

A second common error in question-phrasing is to frame the question at a level of abstraction inappropriate for the class. Students are likely to participate in discussion when they feel that they have an experience or idea that will contribute to the discussion. This means that the discussion questions need to be phrased as problems that are meaningful to the students as well as the instructor. Such questions can be devised more easily if you know something of the students' background. An experiment by Sturgis (1959) showed that knowledge of student background makes a significant difference in a teacher's effectiveness as measured by students' learning.

A third error in raising questions is to ask your question before finding out about the students' problems. Often a good question fails to elicit responses because students are hung up on some prior problem.

Suppose you ask a question and no one answers, or the student simply says, "I don't know." Discouraging as this may be, it should not necessarily be the end of the interaction. Usually the student can respond if the question is rephrased. Perhaps you need to give an example of the problem first, perhaps you need to reformulate a prior question. More often than not you can help the students discover that they are more competent than they thought.

Starting Discussion With a Controversy

Another technique of stimulating discussion is to cause disagreement. Experimental evidence is accumulating to indicate that a certain degree of surprise or uncertainty arouses curiosity, a basic motive for learning (Berlyne, 1960). Some teachers effectively play the role of devil's advocate; others are effective in pointing up differences in point of view.

I have some concerns about the devil's advocate role. I believe that it can be an effective device in getting students to think actively rather than accept the instructor's every sentence as "Truth." Yet it has its risks, the most important of which is that it may create lack of trust in the instructor. Of course, instructors want their students to challenge their ideas, but few want their students to feel they are untrustworthy, lying about their own beliefs.

A second danger in the "devil's advocate" role is that it will be perceived as manipulative. Students may feel (with justification) that the instructor "is just playing games with us—trying to show how smart he or she is and how easily we can be fooled."

A third danger is that the devil's advocate role will be used as a screen to prevent students from ever successfully challenging the instructor. In this use the instructor, whenever the student wins an argument, simply says, "Well I just presented that position to see if you could see its weakness."

Not only are all of these possible problems infuriating for the student, but they maintain a superior-subordinate relationship antithetical to the sort of learning environment that we want. If the best classroom is one in which both students and teacher are learning, a role that provides armor against the instructor's learning is bad.

Yet the devil's advocate role can be effective. Its success depends a good deal upon the spirit with which it is played. My own compromise solution is to make it clear when I'm taking such a role by saying, "Suppose I take the position that ——— " or "Let me play the role of the devil's advocate for a bit."

In any case the instructor should realize that disagreement is not a sign of failure but may be used constructively. When rigid dogmatism interferes with constructive problem solving following a disagreement, the instructor may ask the disagreeing students to switch sides and argue the opposing point of view. Such a technique seems to be effective in developing awareness of the strengths of other positions.

What Can I Do About Nonparticipants?

In most classes some students talk too much and others never volunteer a sentence. What can the teacher do?

Unfortunately, most students are used to being passive recipients in class. To help them become participants I try to create an expectation of participation in the discussion section. You can start to do this in the first meeting of the course by defining the functions of various aspects of the course and explaining why discussion is valuable. In addition to this initial structuring, however, you must continually work to increase the students' awareness of the values of participation. Wise instructors realize that participation is not an end in itself. For many purposes widespread participation may be vital; for others it may be detrimental. But they must try to create a climate in which an important contribution is not lost because the person with the necessary idea did not feel free to express it.

What keeps a student from talking? There are a variety of reasons—boredom, lack of knowledge, general habits of passivity—but most compelling is a fear of being embarrassed. When one is surrounded by strangers, when one does not know how critical these strangers may be, when one is not sure how sound one's idea may be, when one is afraid of stammering or forgetting one's point under the stress of speaking—the safest thing to do is keep quiet.

What can reduce this fear? Getting acquainted is one aid. Once you know that you are among friends, you can risk expressing yourself. If you know that at least one classmate supports your idea, the risk is reduced. For both these reasons the technique of sub-grouping helps; for example, you can ask students to discuss a question in pairs or small groups before asking for general discussion.

Even asking students to take a couple of minutes to write out their answers to a question can help. If a student has already written an answer, the step to speaking the answer is much less than answering a question when asked to answer immediately. Even the shy person will respond when asked, "What did you write?"

Even superficial techniques can help increase participation. Rewarding infrequent contributors at least by a smile helps encourage participation even if the contribution has to be developed or corrected. Calling students by name seems to encourage freer communication. Seating is important too. Rooms with seats in a circle help tremendously.

Getting to know the nonparticipant is also helpful. For example, I have found that it is sometimes helpful to make the first assignment to write a brief life history indicating the student's interests and experiences. These autobiographies help me to gain a better knowledge of each student as an individual, to know what problems or illustrations will be of particular interest to a number of students, and to know whom I can call on for special information. One of the best ways of getting nonparticipants into the discussion is to ask them to contribute in a problem area in which they have special knowledge.

The technique of asking for a student's special knowledge deals directly with the fear of being wrong. No one likes to look foolish, especially in a situation where mistakes may be pounced upon by a teacher or other students. One of the major reasons for the deadliness of a question in which the teacher asks a student to fill in the one right word—such as, "This is an example of what?"—is that it puts the students on the spot. There is an infinity of wrong answers, and obviously the teacher knows the one right answer; so why should the student risk making a mistake when the odds are so much against the student? And even if the answer is obvious, why look like a stooge for the teacher?

One way of putting the student in a more favorable position is to ask general questions that have no wrong answers. For example, you can ask, "How do you feel about this?" or, "How does this look to you?" as a first step in analysis of a problem. The students' feelings or perceptions may not be the same as yours, but as reporters of their own feelings, they can't be challenged as being inaccurate. Although such an approach by no means eliminates anxiety about participation (for an answer involves revealing oneself as a person), it will more often open up discussion that involves the student than questions of fact will.

The Discussion Monopolizer

If you have worked on nonparticipation effectively, the discussion monopolizer is less likely to be a problem, but there will still be classes in which one student talks so much that you and other students become annoyed. As with nonparticipation, one solution is to raise with the class the question of participation in discussion—"Would the class be more effective if participation were more evenly distributed?"

A second technique is to have one or more members of the class act as observers for one or more class periods, reporting back to the class their observations. Perhaps assigning the dominant member to the observer role would help his or her sensitivity.

A direct approach should not be ruled out. Talking to the student individually outside class may be the simplest and most effective solution.

TESTING AND GRADING

Most instructors in colleges with traditional grading systems deplore the emphasis students place upon getting a good grade from the course. Usually instructors attempt to minimize this aspect of the course by stating that the important thing in the course is what the students gain, not what grade they make. Sometimes a few students nod their heads in agreement. While such words are intellectually accepted, motivationally the grade remains the most important aspect of the course for most students. Since grades in large courses are determined to a great degree by scores on tests, the tests are among the most frustrating aspects of the course to many students, and usually arouse a great deal of overt and covert aggression. If teachers, using objective-type tests, attempt to go beyond the usual practice of asking simply for memory of information from the textbook or lectures, they are immediately deluged with the complaint, "These are the most ambiguous tests I have ever taken!"

Reducing Student Aggression

To most beginning teachers the aggression that students direct against them after a test is very disturbing. It is likely to impair the rapport of the instructor with the class and may in some cases actually be a block to learning. Hence, devices for reducing the aggression seem to be worthwhile.

The most obvious solution to the problem is to reduce the frustration involved in taking tests. The most important aid in this area is to emphasize the contribution the course can make to the long-range goals of the students, so that the need of a good grade is not the only motive involved in the situation. Emphasizing the educational and diagnostic value of tests is one application of this principle. Yet, no matter how much the instructor emphasizes long-range goals, the tests are going, in a large measure, to determine the students' goals. Do you want the students to memorize detail? Then give the usual memory-of-details sort of test.

Thus, the first step in constructing a test is to list your goals for the course. Not all goals can be measured by a test. New attitudes and interests, for example, are not measured by classroom achievement tests, but this should not be used as an excuse for avoiding the effort necessary to specify outcomes in measurable terms. Once you have specified objectives you can determine how many test items embody each category of objective. You'll probably be surprised to find out how many of your test items pile up in certain categories.

One way of helping to maintain a balance is to construct a grid, listing objectives along the side of the page and content areas along the top. If you then tally items as you write them, you can monitor the degree to which your test adequately samples the objectives and content desired.

Because some course examinations emphasize recall of facts, many students demand teaching that emphasizes memorization of facts. One student wrote on a slip evaluating me, "This instructor is very interesting and worthwhile, but I have rated him low because he doesn't give us enough facts. The sort of job I get will depend on my grades, and I have little chance of beating other students out for an A unless I can get a couple of pages of notes each period."

Because our objective was not simply memory of facts, but ability to apply principles, the general psychology teaching staff at The University of Michigan attempted to construct items that would measure the students' abilities to apply principles and give them the feeling that application of learning was an important objective of the course. As might be expected, scores on our application items correlated more highly with intelligence as measured by the Otis Test of Mental Ability than did scores on items primarily testing memory (0.41 vs. 0.17). Nevertheless, this correlation was not high enough to indicate that intelligence was the only factor tested, and a semester of psychology does result in gains on these items.

Students may object at first to items requiring them to think, but if you emphasize that the tests will measure the students' abilities to use their knowledge, you can greatly influence their goals in the course. This is indicated by a student's comment we received, "More of the course should be like the tests. They make us apply what we've learned." Marton and Saljo (1976) showed that questions demanding understanding rather than memory of detailed facts resulted in differing styles of study for later tests and better retention.

Student participation in test construction also seems to reduce the aggression occasioned by tests. Explaining the type of test you give, discussing your reasons for using this type, and asking students who would like to contribute items for the next test to submit items helps you tear off some of the cloak of mystery surrounding the test. Actually using some items submitted by students rewards those students who submitted them. Devising questions helps make the students aware of the problem involved in item construction, as well as giving them a good review of subject matter.

Nevertheless, I cannot overemphasize the importance of relating test items to objectives. Admittedly it is more difficult to devise measures of the more complex, higher level objectives. Yet the very effort to do so will, I believe, have an influence on student motivation and learning. Moreover, consideration of these objectives may help you break out of the conventional forms of testing. For example, in my classes in introductory psychology, the desired goals include developing greater curiosity about behavior, awareness of dimensions of behavior that might ordinarily be ignored, and increased ability to describe and analyze behavior objectively. To get at this I have sometimes used a film as a stimulus, with the test questions having to do with the students' reactions to the film; or I have asked students to leave the classroom for fifteen minutes and then report on some interesting behavior they have observed. I have brought in collections of journals and asked them to find an article of interest and to write their reactions to it. I have asked for analyses of newspaper items to get at the degree to which students can read critically. Using materials with somewhat greater apparent relevance to course objectives than typical test items is more fun for the students taking the test—and more fun to grade.

When to Test

Because tests are so important in operationalizing goals and influencing student methods of learning, I like to give a test early in the term—after the third or fourth week of a fourteen-week semester. To reduce the stress, I weight the test very little in determining the final grade, perhaps a third of a comparable hour test given later in the term. Such an early test gets students started, rather than delaying their studying until the conventional midterm examination, and it helps you, or your teaching assistants, to identify problems early while they are still remediable. Thus, this test should demand the style of learning you expect and needs to be constructed carefully, even though its purpose is more motivational and diagnostic than evaluative.

I usually also give midterm and final examinations, but the amount and frequency of tests should depend upon the background of your students. In a freshman course in an area new to students, frequent short tests early in the term facilitate learning, as demonstrated in the Keller Plan. Generally, however, I want to wean students from studying for tests. I want them to become lifelong learners who will be able to evaluate their own learning. This implies less frequent testing as learners become more experienced. It probably also implies questions requiring broader integration and more detailed analysis as the learners advance. For this reason my tests are all cumulative; that is, they cover material previously tested as well as material learned since the last test.

I try so far as possible to give my students a clear conception of what the final exam will be like. They gain from the early tests a sense of the kind of test items I write and I tell them in advance how many multiple-choice, short-answer, and essay items there'll be. Your syllabus can help give the students a beginning sense of what to expect and forms an implicit social contract which you will be ill-advised to break.

Test Construction

This is not the place to engage in an extended discussion of test-construction theory. Let me confess, however, that from the students' point of view, tests and marks are frequently the most important part of the instructor's job. Because of this, these topics deserve some consideration. The instructor who is about to give an examination is in a conflict situation. There are two time-consuming procedures involved in the administration of an examination: the first is the construction of the examination; the second is the grading. Unfortunately, it appears to be generally true that the examinations that are easiest to construct are the most difficult to grade and vice versa. Essay examinations that can be made up in a few minutes require hours to grade. Multiple-choice examinations, which can be constructed by an experienced item builder at the rate of 3–5 items an hour, can be corrected at the rate of about 20–30 seconds for a 60-item test. Short-answer examinations fall somewhere between these two extremes. You will be tempted to use items over and this is feasible if the item represents only a small part of the items in circulation. At one time I tried to maintain security on my tests in order to permit greater re-use of items, but once this is known students develop strategies for creating fraternity files. Thus I now put all my old exams in the library where they are equally accessible to everyone.

Teachers often choose questions solely in terms of class size, using multiple-choice tests for large classes, short-answer questions for medium-sized classes, and essay questions for small classes. Class size is obviously an important factor, but I urge that your educational goals take precedence. This almost always implies use of some essay or other questions requiring analysis, integration, or application.

Essay Tests

Although the short-answer examination is very useful in certain situations, I would recommend that, if possible, you include at least one essay question on examinations in most college courses. Whether or not essay tests are valid measures, experiments indicate that students study more efficiently for essay-type examintions than for objective tests (McClusky, 1934; Monaco, 1977).

Whatever the values of essay tests as evaluation devices, you should also take into consideration their potential educational value. Essay examinations give students practice in organized, creative thinking about a subject and an opportunity to check their thinking against the standards of someone with more experience and ability in the field. Moreover, they may, as we suggested earlier, orient students to work toward objectives beyond memorization of details. Johnson (1975) demonstrated that when marginal comments on earlier tests emphasized creativity, creativity on the final exam was improved.

Finally, if you read the examination yourself (or at least some of them), you get some excellent information about what students are learning. While the teacher can also learn from students' responses to objective tests, the impact on the teacher of what students are learning seems to be greater and more vivid in reading essay tests.

How Long Should the Test Be?

My most frequent error in testing is that I make my tests too long. I estimate about a minute apiece for multiple-choice items, 2–5 minutes for a sentence to paragraph short-answer item and 10–20 minutes for a one-page essay, with half an hour or more for longer essays. While speeded tests are probably as valid as those in which there is ample time, the level of student complaints rises geometrically with the degree of feeling rushed, and there is some evidence that anxious students are especially adversely affected by time pressure.

DISCOURAGEMENT

No matter how effective you are there will be times when things go badly; there will be students who are unhappy; you'll have courses that don't work. Such incidents are depressing; one bad student comment on a rating form seems to stick in our memories much more than a half-dozen glowing testimonials.

Most of us need peer support. The most effective cure for discouragement is to have established relationships with one or more colleagues in which one can talk about teaching—exulting together over new insights and happy outcomes, and providing mutual support and advice when things go badly. Recognizing that even the greatest star doesn't win them all helps some. But one of the most effective strategies for coping with depression is to go beyond recognizing that we're not alone in our misery. While it may sound trite, a series of bad days or dissatisfied students can provide a stimulus for growth. What went wrong? What could make things better? How can we reach the dissatisfied students without losing those who are doing well? These are the sorts of questions which can lead to analysis and constructive changes.

There is danger of over-reacting to one bad day, one bad student, or even one bad semester. Sometimes you and a particular group of students or a particular course just won't click. Most of us are too quick to feel anger, defensiveness, or discouragement at such times.

A PHILOSOPHY OF TEACHING

Explicitly or implicitly each of us is guided by a conception of what teaching should be. You already have some elements of that philosophy as a result of your experiences as a student; other aspects will develop from your experiences in teaching. Putting that philosophy into words provides a helpful background for the many decisions one must make in planning and teaching a course. Here are some tenets that I hold:

1. Education should be guided by a democratic philosophy. This has nothing to do with politico-social doctrine, but is simply a statement of my belief that education is a cooperative enterprise that works best when the student is allowed to contribute to it—when teachers listen and respond.
2. Students are adults. I feel strongly on this point. One of the severest criticisms that can be leveled against North American higher education is that it perpetuates adolescence for another four years. It seems clear that adult behavior is *learned.* If no opportunity to practice adult behavior is allowed, such behavior will not be learned.
3. Instructors can occasionally be wrong. If they are wrong too often, they should not be teaching. If they are never wrong, they belong in heaven, not a college classroom.
4. There are many important goals of college training. Not the least of these is that of increasing the student's motivation and ability to *continue* learning after leaving college.

SOME FINAL WORDS

What can I say about the work of the teacher? Clearly it is not possible to detail in a few summary statements the "best" methods of teaching. Nevertheless, a conclusion that it doesn't make any difference which methods are used is clearly unjustified. Rather, research suggests that decisions about teaching methods do have important consequences in terms of differential achievement of the varying objectives of a course, differential effects upon various types of students, and probable differential effects depending upon other factors such as the instructor, the course content, and the overall "climate" of the institution.

Enjoyment of teaching is important not only for the enthusiasm we communicate to our students, but also in determining interest in continued improvement. Both of these important values are likely to be lost if teaching becomes so routinized and depersonalized that it is no longer fun.

I hope the suggestions I have made contribute to your enjoyment in teaching and to your students' learning.

References

Berlyne, D. E. (1954). A theory of human curiosity. *British Journal of Psychology, 45,* 180–181.

Berlyne, D. E. (1960). *Conflict, arousal, and curiosity.* New York: McGraw-Hill.

Bloom, B. S. (1953). Thought processes in lectures and discussions. *Journal of General Education, 7,* 160–169.

Davis, J. R. (1976). *Teaching strategies for the college classroom.* Boulder, CO: Westview Press.

Hartley, J., & Davies, I. K. (1978). Note-taking: A critical review. *Programmed Learning and Educational Technology, 15,* 207–224.

Johnson, D. M. (1975). Increasing originality on essay examinations in psychology. *Teaching of Psychology, 2,* 99–102.

Katz, D. (1950). *Gestalt psychology.* New York: Ronald Press.

Leith, G. O. M. (1977). Implications of cognitive psychology for the improvement of teaching and learning in universities. *Proceedings of the Third International Conference, Improving University Teaching,* 111–138.

Maier, N. R. F. (1952). *Principles of human relations.* New York: Wiley.

Maier, N. R. F., & Maier, L. A. (1957). An experimental test of the effects of "development" vs. "free" discussion on the quality of group decisions. *Journal of Applied Psychology, 41,* 320–323.

Marton, F., & Saljo, R. (1976). On qualitative differences in learning: II—outcome as a function of the learner's conception of the task. *British Journal of Educational Psychology, 46,* 115–127.

Mayer, R. E., & Greeno, J. G. (1972). Structural differences between learning outcomes produced by different instructional methods. *Journal of Educational Psychology, 63,* 165–173.

McClusky, H. Y. (1934). An experimental comparison of two methods of correcting the outcomes of examination. *School and Society, 40,* 566–568.

Monaco, G. E. (1977). *Inferences as a function of test-expectancy in the classroom.* Kansas State University Psychology Series, KSU-HIPI Report 77–3.

Royer, P. N. (1977). Effects of specificity and position of written instructional objectives on learning from a lecture. *Journal of Educational Psychology, 69,* 40–45.

Solomon, D., Rosenberg, L., & Bezdek, W. E. (1964). Teacher behavior and student learning. *Journal of Educational Psychology, 55,* 23–30.

Snow, R. E., & Peterson, P. L. (1980). Recognizing differences in student aptitudes. In W. J. McKeachie (Ed.), *Learning, cognition, and college teaching* (pp. 1–24). San Francisco: Jossey-Bass.

Sturgis, H. W. (1959). The relationship of the teacher's knowledge of the student's background to the effectiveness of teaching: A study of the extent to which the effectiveness of teaching is related to the teacher's knowledge of the student's background (Unpublished doctoral dissertation, New York University), *Dissertation Abstracts, 19,* No. 11.

Wine, J. (1971). Test anxiety and direction of attention. *Psychological Bulletin, 76,* 92–104.

Much of this material is adapted from my book, *Teaching Tips,* 7th ed., D. C. Heath, 1978.

---

[1]This section is based on my book *Learning, Cognition and College Teaching.* Jossey-Bass, 1980, pp. 25 *et seq.*

---

[2]This technique is one I learned from Norman R. F. Maier, described in his book, *Problem-Solving Discussions and Conferences: Leadership Methods and Skills* (New York: McGraw-Hill, 1963).

5

EVERYTHING YOU ALWAYS WANTED TO KNOW ABOUT RESEARCH BUT WERE AFRAID TO ASK (YOUR ADVISOR)

Mark P. Zanna
University of Waterloo

John M. Darley
Princeton University

An earlier version of this chapter appeared in the *Catalog of Selected Documents in Psychology*. As the title implies, its apparent audience is graduate students. But, as a number of astute readers picked up, it, in fact, had two audiences. At the manifest level the article is addressed to graduate students; at the latent level, however, the audience includes beginning faculty members as well. The implicit message carries advice to the latter on the supervision of graduate students' research projects. In light of the implicit message the chapter is included in the present volume. We and many of our colleagues have found that graduate supervision is facilitated by discussing this chapter with our students. You, too, may want to pass it along.

Over the years, and particularly through supervising graduate students, we have developed a style of conducting research and writing it up that is reasonably successful and shared with many other faculty members. But, as innumerable discussions with our colleagues have revealed, all elements of the system are not always successfully transmitted to our graduate students. Here we propose to set down explicitly this system for ourselves and for our graduate students, in the hope of making all our research tasks easier. We attempt to describe the steps involved in conducting research in social psychology. What we try to do is identify and describe the specific actions to take during the course of a research project. Of course, we cannot provide general answers to all of the questions which might arise. Our best advice is to "learn the ropes" from senior graduate students. A good supportive graduate student culture can be invaluable in acquainting you with such resources as the subject pool (or how one gets subjects), the secretarial pool (or how one gets materials, e.g., questionnaires prepared), and the computer center (or how one gets data analyzed).

We don't propose to talk a great deal about where research ideas come from. They can come from a wide variety of sources. They can be relatively one's own or can come from one's advisor. However, regardless of the exact source of the idea, we find that research goes most successfully and the graduate student learns most when he or she acts as if it is his or her own study. Systematic attention to detail is what makes the difference between merely adequate and really good research and this attention to detail is most evident in students who have taken on the intrinsic motivation implied in the phrase "as if it's your own study." You're not a hired hand. Don't regard yourself as one.

Literature Review

Assume that you have a research hypothesis. Prior to running any subjects you should conduct several kinds of literature reviews. First, you ought to read enough so that you are familiar with the main conceptual references leading up to your study. These will eventually figure in your introduction. Second, and less obvious, you should be aware of studies using methods similar to your own. Some of these studies will appear in your conceptual review; you ought to use the best methods available in the area. In addition, you ought to have a general knowledge of related research areas with an eye to using what might be better and/or more sophisticated techniques than those commonly in use in your own area. Here, a note on graduate student culture is in order. If you have maintained an interest in various areas of psychology and have kept up your contacts with graduate students in other areas, some of these improved methods will naturally come to your attention in your discussions with them. Cognitive psychologists, for example, have a good deal to give to social psychological inquiries. Don't be bound by the set of procedures and methods taken for granted within your particular research area.

THE DESIGN

Design Proposal

Next, work out the experimental design. There are a good many books on experimental design. We now assume that you have read at least one of them and have worked out an experimental design that you think will adequately test your hypothesis. What should you do next? *Consult others*. We can't emphasize enough how valuable it is at various steps to seek other people's reactions to your own ideas. At this point get together a group of graduate students, or faculty and graduate students, and present your design to them. Here the best kind of support they can give you is not undifferentiated enthusiasm, but a close, critical scrutiny of whether your design is the best way of testing your hypothesis. Develop a graduate student culture in which this kind of interaction and support of criticism is normative. As you present your design, don't do so defensively. Don't be so committed to it that you are unwilling to change any elements of it. Instead of playing a combative role during the discussion, take careful notes and try to restate others' points of view so you're sure that you understand them. The ultimate responsibility for the design is yours; you're not obliged to take anybody's comments into account. After the meeting you can go away and think about what you want to do. But be sure you understand what other people were saying so that you can make the best of their comments.

At this point, you should write a brief experimental proposal that will help clarify your ideas. A written proposal will also facilitate more extensive feedback from your advisor and other faculty.

A Brief Aside About Word Processing

Word processors are now available on most mainframe and microcomputers. Such packages can provide valuable assistance in all stages of your research. Also, word processors can facilitate your preparation of teaching materials. If you already know how to type, it is not complicated to learn the new format. As long as the bulk of your material remains the same, you will only have to edit the sections in which changes are made. Furthermore, when word processors are used throughout the course of your research, material from the proposal, protocol and measures can easily be merged into your final manuscript. In other words, those sections of your manuscript that should "write themselves" have already been written (at least, in a related or draft form) and are retained in some form of computer storage.

Word processing systems can exist in various places within the university and at various levels of sophistication. Check to see which are available to you. Finally, we recommend that you take the time to become reasonably comfortable with the system before you enter any important text. Word processors may not increase your efficiency if manuscripts are inadvertently changed or deleted.

Design Problems

Here we outline several difficulties that we have often found in the experimental designs of relatively inexperienced researchers. First, and perhaps foremost, the designs of inexperienced researchers tend to be too complex. This is true at the level of both independent and dependent variables. In the initial stages of research, at least, you should try to keep experimental questions simple and straightforward. Establish a relation between your main independent and dependent variables before you go on to examine the boundary conditions and mediating process(es) in more complicated designs. Also you should consider running a homogenous sample of subjects (e.g., all male or all female subjects) as such a sample is likely to provide a more powerful test of your hypothesis. The generalizability of any effect can always be examined in follow-up studies. In other words, we encourage you to plan programmatic research. All of your questions cannot be answered in a single study. This multiple-experiment strategy is particularly wise for thesis research. Plan to go to your thesis proposal meeting with a sequence of two or three experiments, the first of which has already been completed! Ask yourself: does the design test my experimental hypothesis? Does it do so in the simplest and most direct way possible? We confess that we have a longing for the older experimental designs involving one experimental group and one control group. If you look back over the studies you have read that you think are important, you will discover that most do not have many more groups than that.

Second, many researchers fail to consider alternative explanations for experimental effects at the design stage—that is, *before* they run their experiments! Where possible, these alternatives should be ruled out in advance by design and/or procedure. On the other hand, many interesting studies have been abandoned when a "clean" design cannot be found. Our advice is to establish your effect with a slightly "dirty" design rather than to become paralyzed with alternative explanations. Once you have demonstrated an effect, you can begin the serious, and often difficult, work of ruling out plausible alternatives in follow-up studies.

Third, we recommend that you consider your design in statistical terms. Will the data analyses that follow from it be, first, statistically tractable, and, second, statistically powerful? For example, in analysis of variance terms, do your important effects appear as independent, non-confounded terms in the analysis? Can you structure your major predictions as simple main effects, or are they couched as some sort of higher order interaction prediction which would require a very large number of subjects in order to have any chance of emerging at a conventional level of significance? In short, think through your basic analyses at the design stage and determine that your design will, in fact, allow you to test your hypothesis directly and powerfully.

PILOTING

Let's assume that you have emerged from the above process with an experimental design. (Of course, sometimes you won't. You may have cycled through the above process and perhaps you'll have decided that your original question was one that it is impossible to research at this time, given the current state of development of social psychology.) You may have modified your design. Still, at some point, you ought to have come out of the designing cycle with an experimental design that you are ready to try on the real world. However, you will still have some unanswered questions.

The design you have may be your best "armchair" design but it won't be the best design for actual use. But even though you don't have all your design questions completely answered, it is time to contact reality. It is time to take the plunge and collect some pilot data. (A certain number of graduate students otherwise regarded as quite bright and promising seem to run into trouble at this stage. Having produced a shiny, spotless, experimental design, of which they are rightfully proud, they have a natural reluctance to confront it with the uncertainties of human behavior, where it can be soiled by the actions of subjects. But not even your advisor can bat a thousand; there's no reason to expect that you should.)

Graduate students often seem confused about the purpose of piloting, and we have not found any text that gives an entirely satisfactory set of answers. There are multiple purposes in piloting, and we regard piloting as crucial to the solving of several critical questions. The first one or two pilot subjects should be fellow graduate students who can provide you with reasonably non-threatening feedback on how the various elements of your design construction tie together and also, perhaps mainly, give you information about how you are fulfilling the role of experimenter. Your fellow students will also provide a non-threatening situation so that you can get some practice with this role. Nobody is born an experimenter. Just as you needed some practice before you were comfortable fulfilling your teaching assistant role, you need some practice before you are comfortable as an experimenter. It will help if you think of it in role terms in advance. That is, what will the subjects expect an experimenter to look and to act like? Obviously, they will expect you to be in command of the situation since it is one in which you have the authority. They will expect you to take your research seriously and to respond to the formality of the occasion by dressing in ways that are more formal than the normal ones.

The experimenter and teacher roles may present you with a decision problem that you will need to solve effectively if you are going to be a successful research psychologist. That is, the personal style that you have chosen of dress, of hair length and of general manner may be one with which you are, personally, perfectly comfortable. On analysis, however, you may find it one that causes you difficulties in making contact with some segments of the student population. Undeniably, that style is going to cause you to be less effective in doing research with a wide spectrum of people. College sophomores aside, at various times you will run people drawn from the general population as subjects. How will you appear to them? If your personal style is an extreme one, you have something of a crisis on your hands. You need to ask yourself whether your personal style or appearance is a critical and necessary way of signaling who you are, or if there might not be other ways of effecting the same end.

Some additional comments need to be made about the experimenter role on a more specific level. You need to be comfortable with the way in which you communicate the importance of the research to the subject. Subjects who do not feel that the experimenter is involved in significant research will not feel involved either, and their responses to the experimental stimuli will tend to be random and unpredictable. Some experimenters consciously memorize the speech they give to the subjects, others read it. Others have a script available to cue them but give at least large portions of their speech without referring to it. You will need to work out whichever of these options is comfortable for you. However, a mechanical, stumbling and halting reading of the script is not likely to involve the subject.

Returning now to our main theme: We will assume that by now you have run several of your graduate student colleagues and are on your way to becoming comfortable with your role as experimenter. Next, run your advisor and determine what his or her experience suggests will be useful and necessary in the way of procedure changes. See what suggestions he or she would make about your performance in your role.

After completing these pilots, you are ready to begin piloting actual subjects. The first question to ask is whether the experiment, as you have set it up, is understandable, consistent, and involving for the subjects. If they are confused about what they are to do, or bored by doing it, you will need to restructure the situation. Assuming success at that level, the next point to be checked is the extent to which your independent variable manipulations are affecting your subjects. In your design you are likely to have some checks on your manipulations. How are they working? Here it may make sense to deliberately expand the number of questions you ask about the independent variable manipulations, even if this means that you do not go on with these subjects to take further measures. Understanding the fine grain of how they are affected by the manipulation of the independent variable(s) is well worth your time at this point. Once it is clear that the independent variables are effective, your attention can shift to the main dependent variables. Do the subjects interpret the dependent variable questions as you intended? Piloting gives you a chance to collect data relevant to both the convergent *and* discriminative validity of your dependent, as well as your independent, variables. Don't miss it. Are your data recording systems working adequately? "Data recording systems" need not be taken to mean elaborate apparatus. Even if subjects give their answers verbally, have you set up a data recording page that enables you to systematically and efficiently collect all the relevant information?

Although you will be asking a great many questions of pilot subjects, one of the purposes of piloting is to reduce rather than to expand the number of questions you will finally use. There is a tendency, particularly on the part of inexperienced researchers, to ask too many questions of subjects. Piloting should help you reduce these questions to the few that capture the essence of what you are looking for. There are very few independent variable manipulations that can be ethically carried out on subjects that will survive at full strength through 30 or 40 minutes of wading through a dependent variable questionnaire.

The order of topics to be considered in piloting should now be clear. First, get practice in the role; second, see that the situation is consistent and that it involves the subjects; third, see that the independent variables are successfully and forcefully conveyed; and fourth, see that subjects are responding to the dependent variables in the way that you intended. Only rarely will an experimenter, at least initially, get positive answers to all these questions. Considerable "tuning" of the experiment is important. It is our observation that people who can do this effectively will have consistently better experiments and have more chance of success.

Let's assume that you discover that your independent variables are not coming across very forcefully to the subjects. Do you need to go back to the conceptual drawing board? Is something you consider a unitary variable really a conglomeration of two other variables? The debriefing of pilot subjects should give you considerable information about this. Enlist the assistance of the pilot subjects. Explain that you are beginning a study, that you need their help, and that what you intended by your various manipulations was to create a certain set of perceptions or affects. Did they have those perceptions or experience those affects? What would they suggest that you do differently in order to make your points more clearly? Finally, bring in consultants. Run your graduate student colleagues, particularly those you have not run before, and see what they suggest. Bring in your advisor and other faculty members and see what sort of modifications they would suggest for getting your manipulations across more forcefully. People have different skills. Just as there is likely to be a resident statistics expert, there may well be a faculty member or graduate student who is thought to "have the touch" with these sorts of questions about experimental procedure. Borrow his or her intuitions.

THE EXPERIMENT

Before Running The Experiment

Cycle through this piloting phase until you have solved whatever problems have been turned up by previous piloting. First, stand back from your study. Your design, your manipulations, and your measures have undergone many changes in the course of this piloting. Look back and check that the design, the manipulations, and the measures still connect successfully with the conceptual hypotheses with which you started. Make sure the study is still concerned with what you thought it was, or that it at least concerns something interesting that can be confirmed or disconfirmed in a fairly unequivocal way. Make sure, in other words, that you have not lost your hypotheses, or kept the hypotheses but lost the design. Second, before you begin to run, generate a script of what you're doing, specifying the ways in which you manipulate the independent and measure the dependent variables. Generate, in other words, a complete procedural account of your study in such a way that another person could do an exact replication of it. It is always a good idea to have this archival material so that you can answer questions from other investigators at later points in time. If your research is successful, these questions will probably come. Be prepared for them. Be optimistic; you may be starting a line of research in which it will be important to have follow-up studies. This procedural account will be important for yourself and others when you do so.

Now, you are ready to run the actual subjects. How do you decide when to do this? Here it is important to note one of the misconceptions of the uses of piloting. Pilot testing does not and cannot tell you that you are going to get the experimental results you want. It can tell you that your independent variables seem to be affecting the subjects and that the dependent variables seem to be measuring what you want. But it cannot give you the pattern of the relationship between these two sets of variables. If it could, there would be no point in running the final study. (It should be made clear that our conception of pilot work is not that which sometimes is called a "pilot study," which turns out, on inspection, to be a rather poorly designed version of a study that is followed up on later.)

Make sure that you make a conscious and explicit decision when you leave the pilot phase of your experimentation. Make sure at this point that your manipulations will be done the same way for all the subjects and that you have a formal and effective data recording system. Particularly, make sure now that the randomization of subjects into conditions, which one can treat quite casually throughout the piloting phase, is done formally. Decide in advance, based on power estimates, how many subjects you will need per cell.

How And When To Run The Experiment

It's important to run the actual study before too many shifts occur in the actions of the various people who are running it. Over time one's habits change, slowly and perhaps imperceptibly. If enough time elapses during the course of the experiment some very large changes can occur in the way the subjects are treated. One common experience is that the initial anxiety of running subjects often changes over time to boredom. You'll also want to avoid changes in your subject population. Of course, given that you are going to randomize your subjects into conditions, this is not going to introduce systematic error into your study; however, it may introduce a great deal of noise. Suppose, for instance, that you are doing a conformity study and drawing your subjects from the introductory psychology class. At some point during the term the instructor is going to talk about conformity research. You may have a very aware group of subjects after this happens. But even if your experiment does not concern anything discussed in the introductory psychology class, the students may think it resembles something they have heard discussed. They will then suddenly moderate their behavior accordingly. Finally, an experiment that engages the serious interest of a subject during the relaxed, early part of the term may be regarded very differently, and as much less important, during examination week. In summary: first, we're suggesting that you run quickly; second, if you're running from a student population, run early in the term when tension is less high than it is late in the term. (Remember that similar fluctuations occur in the lives of other subject populations.) So once you begin, run quickly.

Running The Experiment

How can you run quickly in actuality? Here again, the viable graduate student culture, dedicated to helping its members complete research, will be a very important asset to you. When you are running subjects, a good many chores need to be done. The subjects have to be scheduled as to time and place. If they are scheduled long in advance, it is wise to call them and remind them the night before an experiment. But, of course, you may have a very full schedule. If you have helped other graduate students with some of the chores associated with their experiments, they should be willing to help you. For instance, they could call subjects to schedule or remind them for you. Also, you may need other graduate students as second experimenters or to play other roles, such as confederates or observers, in your experiment.

There's a second way of running an experiment quickly that frequently tempts inexperienced experimenters—the idea of running many subjects at once. For instance, you and your fellow graduate students may be leading discussion sections and it may be tempting to think about running your study in one or more of those classes. This thought is most likely to occur when you are doing some sort of paper and pencil study, perhaps an attributional one in which a story is told to subjects and they make inferences about the story participants. However, the ethics of running students who are assembled for classes must be considered. Just as critical, there are severe methodological difficulties in running such groups of subjects. First and most important, your study is likely to lose its impact. A subject who is brought to a novel experimental setting, in which the experimenter takes some care to explain the importance of the study, is likely to take the study more seriously than is a group of people doing a study in surroundings designed for some other purpose. Second, if you run subjects in multiple groups and significant interaction possibilities exist, then your group may constitute an *n* of one. And if each group needs to receive the same experimental treatment, between-group differences other than your experimental variables may account for any differences that you find. Your randomization has not been true. We're all for efficiency, but steps that look like easy ways of achieving it turn out to be traps. Don't run more subjects than you can control during the run and successfully debrief afterward.

Data Analysis

It is our impression that the analysis of data forms the biggest bone of contention between graduate students and their research advisors. In almost every university we have visited, faculty members, when talking to each other about what really concerns them, lament the inability of the current generation of graduate students to analyze data. Nowadays, the students often know more formal techniques of data analysis than the faculty members. Nonetheless, they are, initially, surprisingly poor at it. But, of course, graduate students have a good defense against this accusation. Statistic texts do not train them in the process of data analysis we're talking about, which can be learned only in the context of an actual study. Our main point is that analyses are not completed when the most obvious ones have been done. The following three general notions about data analysis should prove useful: First, analyze your data in more detail than will be presented in your final write-up. Second, conceive of the data analysis as a sequential process. Some initial data analyses may give you initial answers that lead to different subsequent data analyses. Third, conduct the data analyses with due regard for the security of the data and its accuracy.

It is very tempting to input your data and quickly try the one analysis that will indicate whether you reached the magic significance plateau of the .05 level. But before you do this, verify that the data have been input correctly. Although many verification techniques might be suggested, the most effective check requires only a printout of raw data in the format of your coding sheets. A graduate student friend can then help you verify the numbers on an item by item basis. Keep in mind a related concern for data security. Recall horror stories you have heard about graduate students losing their thesis data. It happens. Regardless of the storage medium (cards, disk, or tape) you should always have a backup copy of your data. Cards can easily become damaged and entire data files have been lost. These problems are particularly frequent when microcomputers are used. Since these machines rarely have systems to recover lost data, a backup copy should *always* be made when data is stored on a floppy disk. Carefully document your data analysis so that you can remember what the sometimes obscure notations mean. If the computer doesn't print them out, write the labels of the various variables on the printouts. The general point is this: an inexperienced person analyzing data tends to assume much too short a time frame. In response to editors' queries or your own new perspectives you may be coming back to your data a year or so later. At this time, you may be at a different university and have become used to a different computer system. Label everything so that it is easily understood by you and other people (especially your advisor).

Again, we caution students against a dependence on the computer for statistical analysis. Every faculty member has his or her own horror story about the graduate student who went too quickly to the computer. Ours is this:

A graduate student had done a study in which he predicted an interaction between his two main independent variables. With great enthusiasm, in an otherwise quite sensible presentation, he noted that his computer output indicated that the predicted interaction was highly reliable, and that his hypothesis was strongly supported. Given this apparent confirmation, he went on with some grand plans for future research directions until one of the faculty members present, more experienced about this sort of thing, asked for the interaction to be plotted in terms of the condition means. It turned out that the interaction was significant in the direction exactly opposite to that predicted by the graduate student. His presentation had been a public one; his embarrassment was equally so.

When the data have been collected, don't go immediately to the computer! Record your data on coding sheets first. You may discover something that would otherwise have been obscured by the computer analysis. More important, an advisor who was not raised in the "computer age" will want, at some point, to see the data in this format. Data should be recorded as raw scores to provide sufficient flexibility for your various analyses. Any transformations (e.g., creating indices) can easily be produced afterward by the computer. Also, a data file of raw scores may serve as a backup to other archival storage methods. Some preliminary analyses should then be done "by hand." Try to get a "feel" for your data by plotting frequency distributions or calculating means and, perhaps, some simple non-parametric statistics. (A handy rule of thumb, conveyed to us by one of our statistics professors, is that seven nonoverlapping cases will generally mean a significant difference between two means, regardless of the cell n's!) The analyses produced by the various software packages, while correct to two decimal points, should hold few surprises. The computer should clearly be perceived as an assistant. The order of analyses flows from the design of the study. First, and probably primarily, you are concerned about the differences between your various experimental conditions. The first differences between conditions that you should look at are the checks on your experimental manipulations. The question here is not only do they differ between the experimental conditions, but how strongly do they differ? To what extent did your manipulations create the internal states you desired in the subjects? Second, analyze the main dependent measures. Of course, these are the central analyses you will do. But don't stop here. Look within the experimental groups. Are your between-condition effects stronger for those subjects for whom your checks on the manipulation indicate that your manipulations were most successful? What other analyses are suggested by your openness to what your data are telling you? In what ways can you break out of the analysis of variance mold? Do path or any other causal flow analyses make any sense? If you have sets of questions that you ask of the subjects, do factor or cluster analyses make sense? In all this, you should be paying attention to the experimentwise error rate. Sometimes these analyses should be conceived of as preliminary analyses. For instance, you might be doing an interpersonal attraction study, in which you are interested in looking at the two dimensions of liking and respect. Although you will have generated, say, ten questions about each dimension, you will want to know whether the questions that you expect to hang together will, in fact, do so. Factor analysis or item correlations with total scores are techniques for determining this. Empirically derived factors or scales made up of items that correlate highest with the overall scores can then constitute your main dependent variables.

Recall that the analysis of variance framework answers some but not all of the questions about the data. For instance, it may indicate that an "interaction" term is significant. What this means remains for future analysis. Between which of the various groups do the differences actually lie? Specific comparisons and contrasts done within the general analysis of variance framework can help you to determine this. Consideration needs to be given to whether these comparisons are a priori or a posteriori.

You will be wise to spend considerable time with your computer output before you approach your advisor with it. Advisors are not impressed by graduate students who are not able to explain what they have or who have not organized their material sufficiently to find what they have. We have each grown markedly impatient with graduate students taking up our time by pawing hopelessly through three or four pounds of computer output only to find that the relevant analysis is on computer output back in their office, or worse, is not yet in existence. Do organize to make a presentation to your advisor, and organize it on the grounds we've suggested. Prepare a notebook in which the various data analyses are summarized. For instance, at the top of the page you can cite the question the data analysis answers. (You might cut out the actual questionnaire item, for example, and attach it to the top of the page.) Next, present a table of means; next, the analysis of variance; and, finally, whatever specific comparisons seem appropriate. To overcome a common frustration, also mention in which direction the scale is keyed. What do the high versus the low numbers mean? This becomes particularly relevant when you look at correlations. Horror stories abound about graduate students confidently interpreting a correlation only to discover that one of the variables was keyed in the opposite direction and his or her interpretation was entirely counter to the fact.

Quite seriously, a graduate student who makes an organized presentation of experimental results to his or her faculty advisor, and who has done sufficient supplementary and follow-up analyses to cope with questions raised by the preliminary analyses, is going to give that advisor one of his or her great moments of training and is likely to be regarded more as a colleague than as a student in future dealings. This is one of your best chances to show your competence. Don't let it pass by.

What if you missed the big casino at the .05 level and predictions are not statistically confirmed? In our experience it usually makes sense to modify the experiment and try again. After two attempts, however, your efforts may be better spent on other projects. In any event, before you rerun the experiment, you should try to understand why the first attempt might have failed. Was it because your manipulations did not work strongly enough? Did some dispositional variable of your subjects interfere with your manipulations? Were your dependent variables set up in such a way that they pulled a great deal of variance from subjects within conditions? Were there ceiling or floor effects? In general, what can you learn before you conduct a second version of the study? Assigning people to groups on the basis of their manipulation checks, and retesting the main dependent variables, is one useful way of beginning this sort of analysis. Perhaps, you can conclude from your data that it doesn't make sense to pursue the particular question that you are attempting to test. If your manipulations worked well, your effects didn't come out, and you are convinced that you measured them well, you will need to consider this possibility. But, most usefully, other possibilities may be unearthed that will lead to better second studies.

Oral Presentation Of Your Results

Before you attempt an actual write-up of your results, but after you've discussed them with your advisor, it is useful to present them to a group of interested students and faculty. Many good ideas for the write-up will emerge from this presentation. Discuss with your advisor how to make such a presentation. Recall that you need to motivate listeners about your original research question and why it's interesting. Explain the design. Next, present the results. In every experiment there are two sorts of independent variables: interesting and uninteresting. Uninteresting ones in most studies will include things like sex of subject (unless gender is a variable of interest), order of presentation of stimulus materials, and so on. Your primary experimental manipulations will be the factors of real interest, but do present enough results to justify collapsing across the uninteresting factors. Now present the manipulation checks to demonstrate that your experiment was set up properly. Finally, present the main dependent variables. When you are presenting your material, describe the directions of your effects as well as the significance levels. That is, present means (or other descriptive data) as well as significance levels.

We are describing a relatively informal data presentation to a group of your research colleagues, not a more formal presentation, such as a job talk. We have some elaborate and different suggestions to make about that kind of talk, and we have made them elsewhere (see Darley & Zanna, this volume).

The Write-Up Of The Study

Our first suggestion concerning writing up your research is to read the chapter on this topic by Bem (this volume). After digesting Bem's excellent advice, you might consider our additional suggestions. If you have taken the previous steps we have suggested, many sections of your paper will "write themselves." For instance, you have all the materials available for the method section from the procedural summaries you made when you decided you had finished piloting. The results section can be constructed in the presentational order that we have suggested earlier. The introduction to your article, which is perhaps the third thing to write, is tied to the last step that we suggest in your pilot research, at which point we suggested that you assess exactly what your study was about and whether it still remained important. Here you need simply to tell other people what you decided. Some points to keep in mind about your introductory section: First, the inexperienced writer tends to make it much too long. Given the current pressure on journals, five or six pages is usually all that is possible. Your introduction should begin by setting out the general research area in ordinary language. Next, it should review the important research and scholarship on the issue, and formulate the specific question that will be addressed in the experiment. Next, you can describe in a general way the research that will attack the problem. Make sure in all of this that you have been specific about your experimental hypotheses. Some people conclude the introductory section with an overview of the research design.

The discussion section is the last section that you will do, in terms of both the write-up itself and the development of your research communication skills. Most people find it to be the hardest section to write. We really can't be too specific because that which needs to be dealt with in a discussion section arises from the details of the research. Still, certain general things can be said. First, the two most common errors are (a) to do nothing in the discussion section but restate the data-analytic conclusions; and (b) to have your discussion unrelated to the conclusions arising from the data. Usually, in the normal or prototypic discussion section, it is useful to begin with a summary of your results. We would recommend that the summary not be in terms of the method vocabulary that you have set up. State the results in such a way that ordinary readers can understand them without tedious reference to the details of your procedure. Second, talk about what the results indicate in general for the research area in which they are found. Third (the best authors do this in conjunction with the second point), talk about what limits there are on your conclusions. Inexperienced researchers inevitably claim too much, so be cautious. Any single study inevitably has a whole host of limits. Show an intelligent regard for what these limits mean for your conclusions. Your results may not have come out exactly as planned. How does this affect the conclusions? What problems were inherent in your design and operations that limit what you can say? You ought to be able to flow from this into a discussion of where research might go from this point. That more research is needed, we all know. This in itself is not worth saying unless you can talk about some of the specific questions that such research might address.

Drafts Of The Write-Up

It is a common misconception among graduate students that two drafts of the paper should suffice to see it through successful acceptance by a leading journal. The first draft is written by the graduate student. The student then solicits his or her advisor's comments and makes a second draft which he or she assumes is suitable for submission. (Some students regard this second draft as done largely for reasons of courtesy.) This is all hopelessly wrong. That is, there is a great gap between this expectation and the actual working practices of most successful researchers we know. They are much more likely to do five drafts than two. And they are likely to get a wide variety of critical comments on the drafts, not the least important of which are their own.

We suggest that you write a first draft of the entire paper. (Individual differences exist among advisors here. Some advisors like to see drafts of the various sections of the papers as they are written. We prefer to see the whole paper at once.) The first time you write your first draft, you are likely to transmit it immediately to your advisor, hoping to receive his or her comments by the end of the day. This is not a very good idea. We suggest that you stifle your impulse and let that draft sit for a day or so. Then reread it. Try to read it in a critical fashion. Self-criticism is very difficult, but the people whom we regard as the best authors are capable of it. You will probably find your first draft, on delayed rereading, deficient in organization, solipsistic, and needing to be rewritten almost sentence by sentence. De-center here. Try to read your draft as if it had been written by another person. Try reading it as if you did not know the details of method and procedure. If you did not know these details, how well does it communicate them? Could another person understand your methods and comprehend your research design?

Now, write a second draft. Give this draft to your advisor to look over. (If you want to be crafty, pretend it's your first draft!) Make sure that the draft you give your advisor is a complete one. Graduate students sometimes have idiosyncratic definitions of complete. One of us once got a draft in which all of the tables and figures were omitted, with the assurance from the graduate student that these would follow in a few days. Complete means title, abstract, references, footnotes, tables, figures, and often (in first drafts), appendices. Also, and we can't emphasize this enough, do not let your advisor see a draft of the manuscript until it has been proofread to make sure there are no typographical errors. You don't want your advisor's attention distracted from the true substance of the paper.

Once your advisor has given you comments on your draft, rewrite it. Here again, problems will arise. Frequently, graduate students treat what the advisor takes to be major suggestions for redirection as suggestions for minor revisions only. Try to allow yourself to see the full force of the suggestions for change.

It is useful to think of this draft as a pre-submission draft. At this point, you may need to select an appropriate audience for your manuscript. The preliminary studies in a line of research ought to be written up first for a convention presentation. This forum is particularly useful when studies are not quite publishable in top-ranked journals. If the manuscript is to be a journal article, it is likely to be an American Psychological Association journal. Read the publication manual. This manual contains some remarkably sensible advice on writing, as well as on the formal aspects of the manuscript.

Also read carefully the descriptions of what kind of material is acceptable to the various journals. Editors report that they turn down a remarkably large number of submissions simply on such technical grounds. If the manuscript is your thesis, read various thesis publication manuals and determine which one is in use at your institution.

Next it is useful to check your reference section as well. Make sure that all the references mentioned in the text are present in the reference section. More important, since some of these references may be cited from some months ago, it is useful to reread them. Do the studies you cite make the points for which you are now using them as evidence? Remarkably often, slips occur between the stage at which the references are read and the writing stage. This kind of rechecking is extremely wise.

So far, only you and your advisor have looked at the document. After you incorporate his or her comments, it is a good idea to circulate the paper to people whose constructive criticism you have cultivated. If it's your thesis, this will include your thesis committee. If you have developed a good, supportive graduate culture, it will include other graduate students as well. What you are seeking is constructive criticism. Recall that later your manuscript is going to undergo a rather thorough editorial scrutiny. In order for your friends to be constructive at this time, they must try to assume such a role and try to be genuinely critical of that which is presented to them. You are asking them to criticize it and to make suggestions for improvement. The more thoroughly they do this, the better off you will be.

The wider the variety of perspectives taken by the people giving you criticism, the more useful it is likely to be. It will probably be fairly easy to get criticism from people within your own research area. However, the comments of psychologists working in different research areas can be extremely useful as well. First, they can play the role of ordinary individuals who understand design and statistical considerations. Therefore, they can tell you how well your article communicates to a nonspecialist audience. Second, if their research areas relate to or overlap with your own, they may have some useful content insights. One of your tasks is to talk about the way in which your research relates to psychology in general. Such "outside" readers may be extremely useful in helping you do so.

Our remarks concerning your stance during discussions of the experimental design also apply here. As you get comments on your manuscript, your task is not to refute them and to find them silly but to consider what they suggest regarding changes in your manuscript. These comments will be of different sorts. Some will simply indicate confusions in your write-up whereas others will indicate that you have claimed too much in the way of results. Still others may suggest alternative interpretations of your conclusions which you must consider. Once you've asked somebody to comment on your work, you have committed yourself to taking that person's comments seriously. He or she may have reason to be annoyed if these comments are not incorporated into your future draft. By no means is this a suggestion that you agree with every comment. One useful technique involves getting comments from a set of people and correlating them. In general, if more than one person finds a difficulty, it means a difficulty does, indeed, exist. Different people naturally address different areas of concern in the paper. Some people are most concerned with statistical presentation, others with method, still others with the kind of scholarship shown in the introduction. The more criticism you get, thoughtfully used, the better your final product will be. If the people from whom you are getting comments have had experience in publishing their own articles, you might ask them to give an estimate of what journal you might submit your work to. More experienced people are aware of the traditions and styles of various journals. Use their experience.

In summary, what we have said is to be open to criticism, to be willing to go through a large number of drafts, and to consider a large number of changes in those drafts. Two things are important in enabling you to do so: First, adopt a realistic time frame for this effort; from the completion of data collection to the submission of the article to the journal, "months" is a better range of time than "days." We recall horror stories about graduate students who left a week or ten days between completing the data collection of the experiment and some planned summer vacation, or worse, the onset of a job. The experiment is not "finished" when the subjects are run. The experiment is finished when the write-up is completed. Research on productive psychologists would indicate that the completion time for experiments, defined this way, is more usually measured in years than in months. The problem of leaving sufficient time to complete the work seems particularly acute for graduate students finishing their Ph.D. thesis. One of the most prevalent sources of discomfort on the part of faculty members is the extreme time pressures they feel that graduate students put them under to evaluate their work. Faculty members lead busy lives. Naturally, the most important thing to an all but Ph.D. student is the completion of his or her thesis. Sometimes other job requirements cause it to be less important to the faculty member, regardless of his or her concern for or affection for the student. At one institution we know, three weeks at the end of the academic year are devoted to a hectic set of comprehensive exams for undergraduate seniors, oral exams on their thesis projects, and end of the year course grading. During this time of year faculty members are simply unable to allocate the time needed to give a thesis a serious review. Nonetheless, each year several graduate students allow the months to slip away, present their thesis at this time, and are dismayed when the thesis cannot be processed. Worse, we have seen graduate students who resist making changes in their theses, because to make the changes would require more major retyping than they wish to do or pay for, or would make them miss some thesis completion deadline and delay their degree. Avoid this trap. Particularly try to avoid it on your thesis, but remember this about all papers. There is no point in courting journal rejection by sending a half-thought-through paper to the journal. Inevitably, this means spending more time on the write-up than graduate students initially seem to expect.

The graduate student's second source of resistance to the idea of multiple drafts sometimes comes from his or her anticipation of the sheer mechanical labor involved in typing and retyping the new material (or, in extreme cases, in the unbinding of prematurely bound theses). At many institutions, depending on the way the secretarial support staff works, research projects mutually done with faculty members may be typed by the secretarial group. But don't count on this. Expect to type at least most of the initial sets of drafts yourself. Word processors are particularly valuable in this respect. This is especially true, since you probably ought to recognize that almost every word of your first draft is going to require changing. Very little of what you initially write will survive unchanged into the final version. Take heart, there will be a final draft!

Archival Storage and Visual Presentation

While you are going through various versions of your writeup, time not spent on writing need not be wasted. You will want to collate and make sure that you have available the various kinds of documentary material that are to exist independent of the final write-up. At several points in this paper, we have commented on what some of these documentary materials will be. They include the tabular summaries of the raw data, the complete records of the analyses, and a more detailed methods and procedure section than will appear in the final article. Get them assembled and into an archival site now. In general, arrange for some long-term storage of your research materials. Be particularly careful with the data. Current expectations are that the data ought to be available for five years following the research investigation. Make sure that you will be able to go back to your material, even after a couple of years, and find anything that you need.

In particular, you should investigate the various archival methods available for computer files. While you remain in graduate school, your only concern may be retrieving the data for future reference. Archival storage for this purpose should not present any problems, if you keep careful records of where your data are stored. When your graduate career is over, however, you may wish to take some computer data with you to another university. In this case, you should likely talk with a computer consultant to ensure that the format of your data will be compatible with the computer facilities at the new university.

When writing up your experiment, both while your experimental apparatus is possibly still intact and at earlier points during the study, think about a form of documentation that would be useful if you were giving a formal colloquium on your experiment. Specifically, think about what you may want to photograph. Is your apparatus complicated? A picture usually explains it better than any verbal description. What slides do you want to make of your data? Will some sort of flow diagram of your research design help? In another chapter (Darley & Zanna, this volume) we go into details about an oral presentation, what it entails, and how it is to be prepared for. Here we simply want to make you aware of its possibility. We would suggest that every graduate student learn how to use a 35 mm camera during his or her time at graduate school. Frequently the department owns one or one can be borrowed from a faculty member or another student. (Motion picture or videotape cameras may also be available and may facilitate the presentation of your stimulus material.) Think about the colloquia you have attended. It is likely that the more interesting ones will have used some form of visual or auditory presentation of materials. What can you use? To summarize, while you are preparing your written presentation and materials, recall that an oral presentation of your experiment is also a possibility. Think about what sort of audio-visual and other aids would be useful in this presentation and create them.

A Note On Debriefing And Ethics

Part of the task of the experimenter is to function as a cultural anthropologist, fitting the experiment successfully into the culture of the subject population being run. The pilot subject, then, is as valuable to the experimentalist as the anthropologist's informant is to the anthropologist. The pilot subject is the person who will tell you whether you have successfully achieved all of the little touches that will make your experiment clear and involving to the group that he or she represents.

Both pilot subjects and your regular subjects are valued partners to you in your research efforts; they should leave the experimental situation realizing this. When they leave the experiment they ought to understand completely what the experiment was about, understand the importance of the research question, and understand what contribution they have made to its resolution. Good experimenters tend to leave at least as much time for the debriefing as they do for the actual running of the experiment. Make sure you fit this into both your pilot schedule and actual running schedule.

If your research involves deception, a comprehensive discussion of debriefing can be found in many sources (in particular, see Mills, 1976). In our view, however, subjects should be thoroughly debriefed regardless of whether the experiment involves deception and/or stress. Doing debriefings ourselves, talking to other researchers, and watching people we consider good debriefers in action, it seems to us that a good debriefing is one that involves a great deal of interaction between the subject and the experimenter. Subjects reason things out and participate in their own debriefing. But this does not mean that one ought to go into a debriefing with no idea about what one wants to say. Indeed, you ought to have an outline of all of the points that you wish to cover. The first few times you try a debriefing you perhaps ought to have a script that could carry you through it, leaving places into which the subjects can intrude. Experimenters always have an obligation to debrief their subjects and they should, we suggest, take the opportunity to teach the subjects something about the forms of psychological inquiry. Many experiments are run with subjects drawn from subject pools from psychology classes, and this teaching component was an important consideration in establishing the subject pool in the first place. But whether your subjects come from a subject pool or not, the end of your experiment is a valuable opportunity for teaching the subjects something about psychology. Don't miss it.

Of course you should familiarize yourself with the ethical requirements published by the American Psychological Association. Check within your own university as to whether there is a review committee that is required to evaluate the ethical aspects of all experiments, including your own. Whether or not there is any such formal review, make sure, before you run your study, that you have taken the time to consider it from an ethical point of view. This is facilitated if you discuss it with your advisor, other faculty members, and other graduate students.

One final point: as various radical authors have pointed out, the student is generally in a position of low power. Students get into the habit of thinking that they have so little power that there is no way that they can seriously affect other people and that, therefore, they ought not to worry about what effect their actions might have. But you must realize that if you behave as we have suggested, in an autonomous fashion, you are in a high-power position with respect to the subjects in your experiments. We know some horror stories about graduate students who propose research designs that impose serious stresses and deceptions on subjects. Initially, we questioned the morality of the students and reacted with concern about whether we might not have created a breed of Frankensteins. However, as we have heard these sorts of proposals more frequently, our thinking has changed. There is a great deal of truth in the analysis that students have very little power. One consequence is that they are not in the habit of reviewing their behavior in the terms that more powerful people ought to use. (Recent history suggests that many powerful people are also not in the habit of reviewing their actions in these terms.) Don't create your own scandal, however you would name it. Explicitly think through your study on a human, ethical basis.

Concluding Comments

We have spelled out our image of the "research process" in social psychology. But other people have other images, and it would be helpful to know about them (especially if you are not one of *our* graduate students!). Talk to the faculty you know best at your graduate institution and get their thoughts and advice. There are certain to be many ways in which the picture presented here needs modification. For instance, because of our own backgrounds, we have focused on doing experimental research, primarily in laboratory settings. Some of you will have more applied interests that take you "out of the lab"; some of you will get involved in correlational studies. In any event, we will consider our chapter successful if graduate students (and their advisors) are able to use it as a starting place to discuss modified, or even alternative, images of the day-to-day activities of doing research in social psychology.

ACKNOWLEDGMENTS

We wish to thank numerous individuals who read and commented on previous drafts of the manuscript and, especially, John Hawkins, Jo-Anne McDowell and Shelagh Towson for their editorial advice. An earlier version of this chapter appeared in the *Catalog of Selected Documents in Psychology,* 1980, *10,* 1.

REFERENCE

Mills, J. (1976). A procedure for explaining experiments involving deception. *Personality and Social Psychology Bulletin, 2,* 3–13.

6

ON MANAGING THE FACULTY–GRADUATE STUDENT RESEARCH RELATIONSHIP

Mark P. Zanna
University of Waterloo

John M. Darley
Princeton University

In the preceding chapter we described how to conduct an individual research project. While addressed to a graduate student audience, that chapter also contained advice to faculty on supervising graduate student research. Because this activity is such a significant aspect of a faculty member's responsibilities, it is important to discuss, both explicitly and in more general terms, the management of the faculty-graduate student research relationship. We suggest a model for advising graduate students and describe some of the pitfalls, particularly for new faculty, in establishing a productive research relationship.

Doing research with graduate students, and the relationships that are formed in the process, is one of the most exciting and rewarding aspects of being an academic psychologist. The knowledge that you will interact with bright and creative individuals throughout your teaching career will do a great deal to keep you fresh, motivated, and stimulated with new insights. Training graduate students is the one aspect that makes a professor's career sharply different from almost all other jobs.

Having said this, it must seem as if we are consigning our colleagues who teach at colleges rather than universities to a second class existence. This isn't so. In these colleges, honors majors among the undergraduates often take on many aspects of the graduate student role. They do research studies for their theses, and often there is college money available to pay them to serve as research assistants on faculty research projects. Committed undergraduates often function, in sum, as well as many graduate students. They will know less, on the average, about statistics and experimental design, but may well know more about the theories near and dear to their professor's heart. Faculty working in colleges will need to make some adjustments in the recommendations that follow, but will find that many of them are relevant in their research work with undergraduates.

THE "MODIFIED APPRENTICESHIP" MODEL

Sources of Research Ideas in Faculty—Student Collaborations

The central issue to be dealt with initially by a faculty member is how to identify a research project on which the graduate student will work. On the one hand, it might be sensible to have the faculty advisor wait until the graduate student brings forward a research proposal of his or her own. Alternatively, the graduate student might be assigned to a faculty advisor to work on the next experiment in the faculty member's research grant. We would suggest that neither of these two options is sensible. One is too unrealistic; the other too authoritarian. Instead we suggest a model for advising graduate students, the "modified apprenticeship" model, that lies somewhere between these two extreme alternatives.

When a graduate student begins graduate school, he or she is either explicitly matched with a faculty advisor or asked to seek one out. When we are paired with or approached by a graduate student, we certainly attempt to discover that graduate student's interests, but we also are quite firm in giving that graduate student an initial project that derives from our own research interests. In that way, the graduate student gets the benefit of our time and expertise in an area that we know well and begins early in his or her graduate career to learn the multiple tasks of doing research.

Does this mean we "hand" the graduate student a project? Not exactly. A graduate student is not a research assistant. Instead we give a graduate student an idea with, perhaps, some thoughts about how that idea might be turned into a study. The graduate student does background reading, develops some ideas of his or her own, and together we design the study. While we have thought about a design and procedure beforehand, the graduate student is genuinely engaged in working with us on it, and, in fact, his or her participation at this level almost invariably makes the study better. Graduate students have often thought of ingenious solutions to problems. Also it is useful for them to structure the researcher-subject interactions, since they will eventually play the role of researcher. They will have created an experimenter's "personality" with which they can be comfortable.

The Number of Research Directions Possible

It is our goal to have a beginning graduate student gathering data by the end of the first term or the beginning of the second term. However, during this time, we also begin to discuss with graduate students research that derives from their own interests. We find it very important for graduate students to be working simultaneously on two lines of research. If one line of research bogs down, the other may be productive and the student may thus be shielded from feeling anxious and/or depressed about his or her research abilities. If one line of research gets held up while waiting for the availability of subjects, ethics committee clearance, or for a number of other reasons, the second line of research provides something else on which to work. As we've indicated, the first line of research usually stems from our interests, and we think it ought to be started quite quickly. The second line of research stems more from the interests of the graduate student, and the graduate student can be doing the reading and developing the research ideas while also working on the first line of research. Typically, the graduate student's M.A. thesis comes from the first line of research. In fact, the M.A. thesis often reports the first study done. If all goes well, the Ph.D. thesis comes from the second, more independent line of research developed by the graduate student. Incidentally, this latter line may change several times in the course of the graduate student's career. Students need not stick with initial ideas that prove experimentally or theoretically intractable. What this means is the relationship between a graduate student and a faculty member begins, as it must, unequally, but shifts toward a more equal status relationship, that of research colleague, by the end of the graduate student's career.

When we suggest that a graduate student should have an independent line of research, we do not mean that the research line must necessarily be divorced entirely from the research interests of the faculty advisor. In fact, particularly in the beginning of the faculty member's career, advising will probably go better if that line is connected to one or more of the faculty member's interests. The simple point is, it should be a line of research, a set of studies, that the graduate student takes the lead in developing. When we say the first line of research should stem from the faculty member's interests, we do not mean to deny the possibility of what often happens: the graduate student sees the need for and designs a second research study (or set of studies) that might not have been conceived of by the graduate advisor. If we are playing our advising role properly, the graduate student can move that line of research onward.

Working With Other Faculty

We encourage our students to work with at least one other faculty member. In the graduate programs that seem to us to be the most exciting, collaboration develops between faculty members and graduate students, so that various teams of individuals are carrying out various research projects. When possible, we sometimes try to facilitate this by having another faculty member designated as a second, or backup, advisor for each graduate student. The backup advisor can play various useful roles such as friendly critic or devil's advocate.

A backup advisor provides a second source of advice for the graduate student. For this system to work best, faculty members ought to be willing to play this role for each other's students. Thus, all faculty gain the benefits of having another advisor for their students, but must, in turn, be willing to serve as backup advisor for other faculty as well. This role proves particularly valuable when a faculty member goes away on leave; the backup advisor, who is well aware of the graduate student's research progress, can quite easily step in as advisor.

There is another reason for our recommendation of a system in which students have a chance to work with one or more advisors. A graduate student who works only with a young, relatively unknown faculty member, and does not take the chance to work with a more senior, more internationally known faculty member, is acquiring a severe handicap on the job market. Therefore a system in which graduate students know that they have a chance to rotate advisors is, in fact, a system that makes it possible for them to choose to begin working with a younger faculty member. Otherwise they would have to choose against the beginning faculty member.

How Many Students to Advise?

The modified apprenticeship system we have described has an important limit. We have found it works best when a faculty member has three or at most four graduate students to advise. In fact, we would be able to cope with three or four students only if the graduate students were at different stages of their Ph.D. careers. In this way the more senior graduate students can "show the ropes" to the newer graduate students and pass on some of their skills to those graduate students. This not only helps the faculty member and the junior graduate students, it also helps the senior graduate students learn some of the skills involved in training students to do research. In universities in which undergraduates do honors theses, many faculty members may also involve their graduate students in the supervision of undergraduate theses. The graduate student benefits from this opportunity to teach senior level undergraduates as well. This can be overdone, however. While a graduate student may help with the supervision of an independent honors thesis, especially if it is in an area of his or her own research expertise, the honors undergraduate may resent being advised primarily, or even solely, by a graduate student.

We might clarify for beginning faculty the implications of what we are saying. In spite of the irrepressible desire to begin rapidly and to get a great deal of research completed, we would advise the beginning faculty member not to take on three first-year graduate students. Far better to take on graduate students at the rate of one a year; some of the training done with the senior graduate students can subsequently be passed along by them to the younger people. Don't overload.

DIFFICULTIES OF ADVISING GRADUATE STUDENTS

The Psychological Situation of the New Faculty Member

This is our vision of how the graduate student-faculty advising relationship would work in an ideal situation. But there are many ways in which the relationship can go wrong. Since many of the difficulties will certainly spring from the complex personal relationships that develop between the new faculty member and the student, we need to analyze the particularly difficult transition that is being made by the new faculty member. It is the source of a number of these complexities.

As the new faculty member moves to his or her new teaching setting, the individual is likely to experience a great deal of situationally induced loneliness as well as a good deal of ambiguity about the demands to be made on him or her. That ambiguity produces a good deal of additional anxiety. Because of their age and lifestyle similarities, new faculty members are often drawn to graduate students as potential friends. Yet because of the recently acquired status of the faculty member, a gap is created which is not only difficult, but also inadvisable, to bridge.

Many of the problems encountered by new faculty in establishing a professional research relationship with graduate students stem from this tendency to look to that group for friendships. The necessary but sad truth that the new faculty member must recognize is that he or she has taken a place on the opposite side of the desk from the graduate student. This is enormously hard to appreciate because a mere two or three days earlier the new faculty member was him- or herself a graduate student. Nonetheless, the beginning faculty member must recognize that the essence of his or her job is to teach and train graduate students and in so doing he or she must advise, direct and *evaluate* graduate students. The responsibility to sanction a student, e.g., to place a student on probation, is one responsibility that we all hope will occur rarely. Nonetheless, evaluation, both positive and negative, is one of the essential components of the relationship between faculty and students, and it is one that almost always is underestimated by beginning faculty. Following are some of the classic manifestations of the problem:

A faculty member may become involved in a "hand holding" relationship with graduate students, giving advice on their personal lives. More than giving advice, he or she may be drawn into giving sympathy, even "therapy." Not only does this take an emotional toll on the new faculty member, it can also consume an inordinate amount of time. (Recall the comments about discretionary time made in the Taylor and Martin chapter.) Time spent providing therapy is time not spent in providing graduate education. More to the point, time spent in this way implicitly, but absolutely, undermines the essential evaluative nature of the relationship between faculty and student. (Although we cannot expand on it here, it is important to point out an obvious fact: this trap may be harder to avoid for female or minority faculty members, if only because such faculty are often in "short supply" and are expected to be more nurturant, perhaps by "nature" or by virtue of the circumstances, e.g., "We've got to stick together.")

If a new faculty member is perceived by other faculty members as not having an appropriately role-limited relationship with graduate students, then that faculty member is limiting his or her effectiveness as an advocate for graduate students. Every faculty member will, at some time, want to be an advocate for a particular graduate student; will want to convince other faculty that this student has talents and skills and potential that other faculty may not have glimpsed. Further, most faculty will be drawn, at some time, into mediating a conflict between another faculty member and a graduate student. Neither task is very effectively accomplished by any faculty member who is seen by other faculty as having an inappropriately personal relationship with the graduate student in question. The faculty member's ties to the graduate student provide an all-too-ready alternative explanation for the advocacy. Thus, exactly because the junior faculty member will want to act as an advocate and, possibly, a mediator, it is advisable for junior faculty to establish appropriately structured relationships with graduate students from the beginning.

Finally, it is difficult for the beginning faculty member who identifies closely with a graduate student to do academic advising. For example, it is sometimes necessary for a faculty member to explain to a graduate student that although he or she has been struggling under vast and real personal problems, nonetheless, the impact of his or her lack of academic progress is such that he or she must be put on academic probation or leave graduate school. It is also sometimes necessary to advise a graduate student that, notwithstanding his or her conflict with a particular faculty member, the graduate student has been assigned a teaching assistantship with that faculty member or that the faculty member will be a member of the student's thesis committee. A relationship with a graduate student that makes it difficult to carry out any of these communications or, worse, makes the faculty member appear to have betrayed the student, is symptomatic of role confusion on the part of the graduate student and, most certainly, the new faculty member.

Prototypical Examples

We will illustrate several of the possible beginnings of disaster. When a new faculty member arrives at the institution, he or she is likely to be subject to very flattering approaches from a number of mid-career graduate students who each seek to have the faculty member work with them in various ways. Many acute problems lie herein. If the graduate student has not successfully met the demands of the existing faculty, he or she may have no one to work with. Facing the necessity to work out some sort of thesis project, such a student is often somewhat desperate to find a faculty advisor and is willing, often unconsciously, to be very seductive to do so.

A related case is one we might label the "rescue mission." Some graduate students who have many talents and very well-developed interest patterns, may be "misfits" in the graduate program which a new faculty member joins. That is, while in a "perfect world," there ought to be a faculty member willing to work with those talents on the problems in which the graduate student is interested, in fact, no such faculty member exists. This may be particularly poignant for the new faculty member who may recall graduate students within his or her own graduate program who were similarly "misfitted." Moreover, feeling a commitment to the success of this graduate program, the new faculty may see this as a waste of talents of the graduate student. Given these factors and given a belief that there is a general obligation of the "system" to help the graduate student, the new faculty member may feel that the obligation rests with him or herself. Such an obligation or commitment, we should add, could last several years!

Such obligations are not unequivocal and it is frequently unwise for the new faculty member to take responsibility for advising graduate students in such circumstances. Let us add a personal note. Both of us, when we began teaching, took on graduate students because we were subject to the feelings we have described above. Many of our colleagues report to us that they also have done the same thing. The simple fact of the matter is that it is very difficult to say no, especially when one is a new faculty member. Nevertheless, and interestingly, most of us report that we acted very differently when we moved to our second teaching institution or grew more experienced in our first. Given the second chance, we tended to be very cautious about taking responsibility for students who had been admitted some years before we arrived, or had bounced around among several other advisors.

We have suggested that there are highly idealistic reasons for supervising graduate students. Let us now suggest that there are some less idealistic ones as well. All of us have an image of how much work we could get done on our own research if we could simply have another pair of hands helping with the task. That too can be a motivation for taking on graduate students. We think this is a rather poor motivation. Almost every experienced graduate advisor we know would suggest that advising graduate students is not an efficient way of getting one's own work done. While this may be less true when a student is just beginning graduate school, it certainly becomes more and more true as the graduate student gets nearer to doing his or her Ph.D. thesis. This is as it should be, since it is appropriate that graduate students work on their own problems for their theses. For these reasons, both structural and personal, a number of difficulties lie in wait for the beginning faculty member establishing relationships with graduate students, particularly graduate students who are already some distance through the graduate program.

These problems are exacerbated when a new faculty member is not merely friendly with but, in fact, a close friend of a graduate student. Not only will difficulties arise from the disproportionate amount of power possessed by the faculty member, but such friendships can generate additional problems among both the graduate students and faculty colleagues. Some graduate students, concerned about the distribution of resources and entitlements within the graduate student population, may feel that a faculty member's friendship gives one of their peers an unfair advantage. Faculty colleagues may fear that material confidential to the faculty community will be transmitted to the graduate student community. The ambiguous role of the junior faculty member may also confuse other faculty about one's unequivocal commitment to faculty member status. They also may not know how to treat, or interact with, the graduate student friend.

Partial Solutions to the Problem

Our first and, perhaps, best advice is straightforward: maintain a professional distance from the graduate students. While it is appropriate to discuss professional ambitions and personal matters insofar as they affect the graduate student's training and alternate job preferences, it is inappropriate to dwell on discussions of personal matters if they provide what may become a defense against doing adequate work in graduate school. Short of medical and life-threatening emergencies, it is most important for graduate students in the 1980s to keep their careers on track. Should a graduate student have serious personal or psychological problems, the best thing a faculty member can do is advise the student to seek professional help.

One other consideration ought to be kept in mind and will naturally limit interactions with graduate students: the effective management and allocation of time. All of us are prone to make commitments to graduate students that are not completely warranted. At the very least, we can recognize that this ought to limit taking on other commitments. While a commitment to an occasional rescue mission may be appropriate and even honorable, a sequence of such commitments signals an inappropriate orientation in a faculty member.

In any event, *before* taking on a graduate student it is wise to discuss the student's past performance with relevant faculty members, consult the student's records and files and, if you have any misgivings whatsoever, commit yourself only to a "trial period," during which time the student knows he or she must demonstrate an ability and motivation to progress on some research project.

Testing a Student's Research Ideas

In order to help you decide whether to commit yourself to advising a graduate student, especially a mid-career student, you might also ask the student the following six questions (developed by a colleague for just such a decision):

1. "What is it you're interested in doing/finding out?" (i.e. "What's the big question?")
2. "Why are you interested in doing this?" (i.e. "What's so important about this topic/question?")
3. "How does what you're interested in doing relate to what is already known?" (i.e. "What does the literature tell us?")
4. "How does this research differ from and/or extend previous research?" (i.e. "What knowledge is likely to result?")
5. "How are you going to do this?" (i.e. "What's the method and, possibly, the design?")
6. "What do you expect to find?" (i.e. "What are the hypothesized results?")

By posing these questions, one can assess the amount and, more importantly, the quality of thought that has gone into the research being proposed by the graduate student. Students who do not "pass this test" are not likely to convince our colleague to be their advisor (or even, for that matter, to serve as a member of their thesis committee).

Finally, prior to taking on a Ph.D. student it makes sense to serve on a few M.A. and Ph.D. thesis committees to gain a perspective on what is and what is not considered acceptable as a thesis, how much direction it is normative for the advisor and committee members to give, and so on. We recommend that new faculty members do this as soon as possible.

Danger Signals

Let us try and mark certain danger signals for any new faculty member.

1. If you find you are consistently committing yourself to advising graduate students on Ph.D. theses that are outside your own area of expertise, watch out. You do not have the time to learn these areas, and you are unrealistic if you think that you can successfully advise people without knowing the areas. You are saying yes too often and run the risk of spreading yourself too thin.
2. If, in your first year, you find yourself advising a host of students who were admitted before your arrival, beware! If these students are genuinely going to do work in your interest area, that is one thing; if they are doing work in a scattered range of fields, that is a problem. You certainly run the risk of being perceived as the person on whom to "dump" problematic graduate students and if your time is taken up with senior students, you won't be able to admit students for whose entire graduate education you will be responsible.
3. If you find yourself advising a number of students, and are disappointed by the rate at which those students are progressing toward their theses, you may need to examine what's going on! You may have committed yourself to a number of students who are highly competent excuse-givers, but who are not equally competent graduate students.
4. Finally, if you find yourself, out of a sense of duty, advising a number of students from whom you are not getting any enjoyment, any intellectual stimulation, or any personal benefit, something is wrong. You may be overestimating your resources, overestimating your available time and, importantly, overestimating your skills and knowledge in the areas outside your own expertise. Advising students is a major responsibility which you should not take lightly; but it should also be a challenging and stimulating activity.

Avoiding Difficulties

We recognize that the above advice may appear to be inordinately dispassionate. However, there are many strategies that will allow junior faculty members to become less deeply embroiled in the lives of the graduate students in their departments or programs. First, we would suggest that junior faculty members consciously develop professional and personal relationships with individuals, other than graduate students, who share the faculty members' concerns. Beginning faculty members might recall their own graduate student peers. Although relationships with these individuals may have been competitive in the last year of graduate school, chances are that at least some of these individuals are experiencing many of the same feelings of isolation and uncertainty. As the telephone company likes to remind us, these friends may be but a phone call away.

Second, one can seek friendships with other assistant professors in other departments within the university. This is sometimes quite difficult to do because departments frequently stay very much to themselves. Still, with a certain amount of effort one can turn up some very interesting people with whom one can talk about mutual anxieties and concerns and who may become friends.

In this chapter we have discussed the conduct of advising graduate student research. Doubtless there are other, equally effective models. Since this is one of the central aspects of a faculty member's professional life, we urge beginning faculty members to develop their own model for graduate training and to strive to make it work. We hope that by discussing problems often encountered by beginning faculty in establishing research relationships with their graduate students, we will have helped the following generations of graduate advisors adapt to their new roles.

ACKNOWLEDGMENTS

We wish to thank Shelley Hymel, Louise Kidder, Arie Kruglanski, Ken Rubin, and Betsy Zanna who read and commented on previous drafts of the chapter.

7

RESEARCH GRANTS: A PRACTICAL GUIDE

Robert A. Baron
Purdue University

Stop 50 people at random on the street and whisper the following words into their ears: "NSF; NIMH; NICHD; ONR . . ." How will they react? Probably, with blank stares and looks of total bewilderment. To most, these terms will simply be so much "verbal salad." But now, perform the same task with 50 psychologists. Here, you are almost certain to evoke very different reactions. Eyes will open wide—and may fill with tears of love or nostalgia; voices will tremble as they utter words of endearment (or shake with anger as they mutter epithets of resentment!); and arms may reach out in a gesture of longing and tender desire. The reason for such powerful reactions (which I believe I have only slightly exaggerated) is straightforward: the organizations named above—prosaic as they are—have been the major source of federal support for psychological research during the past three decades. To many members of our field, therefore, they have acquired an almost mystical meaning. Indeed, they are often viewed as something akin to "La Dolce Vita," the pot of gold at the end of the rainbow, and buried treasure all rolled up onto one!

Unfortunately, as you probably already know, these sources of support—meager though they have been—have recently been reduced even more. Massive cuts have befallen many programs that have traditionally provided funds for projects in psychology. For example, the program I headed at NSF from 1979 through 1981 (Social and Developmental Psychology) was slashed from $3.4 million in fiscal 1979, to only $800,000 in fiscal 1982! Given these massive cuts, one might argue that a chapter such as this—which seeks to offer practical advice on maximizing one's chances in the grant support system—now borders on being an exercise in futility. After all, if there are now virtually no grants, why bother to learn how the system works, and how to compete within it effectively? My answer to such remarks is as follows. Certainly, we *have* suffered massive reductions in the level of support for our field. But my two years in Washington taught me that virtually *everything* connected with the federal government functions in cycles. At the moment, we are badly out of favor and must fight what amounts to defensive, rear-guard action. In the future, though, this situation may well change greatly, and permit further infusions of support into our field. I am encouraged in this respect by the fact that the basic administrative structure underlying support for psychology is still largely intact at each of the major granting agencies mentioned above. Thus, for example, at NSF, Social and Developmental Psychology still exists as a separate program—despite the fact that it has virtually no funds to distribute. Should the situation change, it stands ready and able to resume full-scale operations.

With these thoughts in mind, I have prepared the following comments on federal grants. Basically, they represent my attempt to summarize some key facts about the granting process—facts I wish *I* had known (or at least grasped more fully) before submitting some of my own proposals. As you will soon see, my remarks touch on a wide range of issues—everything from why it is important to seek grants, plus an overview of the granting system and how it operates, through comments on budgets, the mechanics of applying, and some common pitfalls that trap many otherwise worthy proposals.

GETTING A GRANT: WHY IT'S IMPORTANT

In recent years, only about 10%-20% of all proposals in psychology submitted to federal agencies could be funded. Given these devastating odds, why should researchers bother? In short, why should they invest many hours of hard work in an undertaking that seems destined to fail? Actually, there are several strong and persuasive reasons for doing so. The ones I view as most important are summarized below.

Grants Support Research

The most obvious of these, of course, is this: without a research grant, many lines of investigation simply can't be pursued. Sophisticated new equipment, substantial amounts of computer time for data analysis, payments to subjects, animal care, salaries to skilled assistants—these and other costs often cannot be covered by an individual's department. Thus, in many instances, grants are a necessity, *not* a luxury. Without the financial assistance they provide, valuable lines of study cannot be carried to completion.

Grants Support Students

A second important reason for seeking outside research support involves the future of our field. Traditionally, funds provided by research grants have made a substantial contribution to the support and training of graduate students. In their absence, the number of students in a given program must usually be reduced. Further, those remaining find it necessary to obtain support through teaching, counseling, or other duties. While these are certainly valuable, they do not contribute to the development of research-related skills—ones most psychologists view as central to excellent graduate education. In sum, it is important for individual scientists to obtain research grants for a simple but basic reason: by doing so, they contribute to the training of future generations of researchers, and so to the continued existence and vigor of our field.

Grants Support Departments and Universities

Third, grants also contribute to the health and well-being of recipients' academic departments and universities. The overhead (or indirect costs) on research grants is an important source of funds for many universities. Indeed, without it, they would find it necessary to curtail many of their programs, especially ones relating to graduate education. Thus, grants are important in this regard, too.

Grants Aid the Careers of Individual Researchers

Finally, research grants are good for researchers, as well as their departments or universities. When an individual receives a grant, it often provides funds that free her or him from other duties. As a result, the investigator has more time to devote to research than would otherwise be true. In addition, receiving an award of outside funds contributes to the status and professional standing of recipients. Research grants are viewed as an official "stamp of approval" from one's colleagues—a concrete indication that the investigator's research is perceived as valuable and important by the research community. In this respect, then, receiving a grant can contribute to a researcher's future career.

To summarize: research grants are of substantial benefits to recipients' fields, their students, their departments, and also to their own careers. Thus, they permit the persons who receive them to satisfy both important altruistic motives, and more personal ones as well. This is a rare combination of benefits indeed, and one well worth seeking even in the face of the daunting odds outlined above.

THE REVIEW PROCESS: HOW IT WORKS

Grant proposals are truly labors of love. Much hard work, creativity, and concern go into their preparation. In view of this tremendous investment, each principal investigator wishes to feel that his or her proposal, once received, will be evaluated in as fair and impartial a manner as possible. Is this actually the case? Having spent two years at NSF overseeing this process, I can honestly answer *yes*. The review system is just about as fair as any human endeavor charged with such a complex task could be. Perhaps the best way of illustrating this fact is that of briefly describing this process for you.

The Review Process: A Summary

At the heart of the system followed at NSF (and at most other granting agencies, too) is a central idea: *peer review*. Briefly, this approach suggests that all proposals should be evaluated by an investigator's peers—other scientists possessing sufficient expertise and knowledge to judge its merits fairly. At NSF, implementation of this guiding principle involves three major steps.

First, all proposals are sent for review to at *least* six *ad hoc consultants*. These are individuals chosen by the director of a given program (the Program Director), and the criteria for selecting such consultants are clear. First, they should be individuals with expertise in the content area of the proposal. Second, they should be persons *without* any personal ax to grind, insofar as the specific proposal is concerned. For example, they should *not* be persons currently embroiled in a scientific controversy with the principal investigator. Nor should they be students of this person, or one of her or his mentors. The goal, then, is that of attaining expert input on the proposal from a group of knowledgeable scientists who can comment on its relative strengths and merits in as dispassionate a manner as possible. Unfortunately, it is relatively rare for all six consultants to respond. Some are too busy; others may be away from the office at the time the review is needed; and still others may have connections to the principal investigator unknown to the Program Director, and may feel that it is inappropriate for them to serve as reviewers. In any case, ad hoc consultants who *do* respond serve as one major source of peer input about each proposal.

Second, proposals are sent for evaluation to members of a standing *advisory panel*. The members of this panel are all active and highly regarded scientists—persons whose judgment is widely respected in the field. At NSF, the Social and Developmental Psychology panel (or *advisory subcommittee*, as it is officially known) consists of six persons:

four social psychologists and two developmental psychologists. These persons (who serve as panel members for 2–3 years) have two major duties. First, they provide written evaluations of proposals submitted to the Program. Second, they attend special meetings (usually held in Washington) at which all proposals received within a specific time period are discussed and evaluated. All panel members receive all proposals, and examine each of these documents. However, the Program Director selects three members to devote special attention to each proposal. These are the individuals whose own interests and expertise seem most closely related to the content area of such proposals.

Third, all proposals are discussed fully by the entire advisory panel during the meetings mentioned above. These meetings take place three times a year, and are often grueling affairs. Indeed, they often begin before 8:30 A.M., and continue until past 6:00 P.M. on each of two consecutive days. Clearly, then, the field owes a great debt of gratitude to panel members for their generous and invaluable service.

During panel meetings, all reviews of each proposal—those provided by ad hoc consultants and those provided by panel members themselves—are discussed and considered. On the basis of this information, plus additional points raised during the discussion, those proposals deemed most meritorious are selected. These are then recommended for support by the Program Director. (Incidentally, the task of recommending a given project for support is far from simple. It involves preparation of several documents that point out the major purpose of the planned research, and fully explain its scientific value.)

In sum, each proposal is considered by a number of peer scientists—both ad hoc consultants and members of the standing advisory subcommittee. The feedback provided by these knowledgeable individuals, plus the often lively give-and-take during panel meetings assures that the principle of peer review is an actual as well as an ideal *modus operandi* at NSF. (And let me hasten to add that while the details of the process differ across various granting agencies, the overall approach and goals remain very much the same.)

The Peer Review System: Some Potential Sources of "Noise"

As I hope the above description indicates, the peer review system used by NSF and other granting agencies really works: it assures that each proposal is evaluated by scientists knowledgeable in the area it considers. In general, then, the system is an eminently fair and reasonable one. But this is not to say that it is perfect. As is true of any communication network among human beings, potential sources of "noise" exist, and should be carefully considered. I would like to mention several of these here, along with concrete steps principal investigators can take to minimize their impact.

First, it is sometimes the case that a proposal falls along the boundary between two adjoining fields (or even areas within a field). For example, it may be concerned with some aspect of social perception, but also draw heavily on (and have implications for) basic aspects of cognition. Or, it might focus on some aspect of group functioning, but also have links to the law and legal processes. In most cases of this type, the joint nature of the proposal will be recognized by the Program Director, and appropriate steps taken. (For example, the proposal may be reviewed jointly by two or more programs; or the director of the program to which it is submitted may seek recommendations for ad hoc reviewers from other program officers.) But remember: program directors are only human. Thus, the possibility exists that they will overlook such connections. The moral for principal investigators, therefore, is clear: *if your proposal does fall on or near the boundary of two fields, call this fact to the attention of the appropriate person at the agency to which you are submitting*. It may well be noticed even if you don't intervene, but why take even the small chance that it will not?

Second, some proposals are concerned with new and innovative areas of research—ones currently being investigated by a small number of scientists. And others deal with topics that are not the focus of a great deal of current interest. In such cases, it may be difficult for the program officer—no matter how conscientious or well-read she or he is—to identify six or more expert ad hoc consultants. I certainly experienced this problem myself on many occasions. (Indeed, I vividly recall the painful headaches brought on by the frustration of attempting to identify the fifth or sixth consultant for some proposals!) In cases of this type, a program director can turn to several sources for help—panel members, other officers at the granting agency. But one key source of assistance may lie with the principal investigators themselves. At NSF, the Social and Developmental Psychology program specifically requests that investigators suggest the names of up to six persons qualified to review their work. And these suggestions *are* used. (I made it a standard practice to select one or two reviewers from this list for each proposal.) Much to my surprise, though, many investigators failed to respond to this appeal for help. Perhaps they believed that the offer was too good to be true—that we really wouldn't use the names they provided. Or perhaps they felt inhibited about recommending friends and personal acquaintances as reviewers. Whatever the reason, they missed a good opportunity to have some impact upon the review process for their proposals. My basic advice, then, is as follows: don't let this happen to *you*. When you submit a proposal, check with the administrative person in charge to determine whether he or she would appreciate suggestions about potential reviewers. And if this is the case, *be sure to provide such input promptly.* This is especially important if your proposal deals with a new area of research, or one that is currently less than torrid. But it may be useful in other instances as well. Basically, this is one of those rare cases in which life may allow you to have your cake and eat it too. The information you supply will assist the program officer with whom you deal; and there is a good chance it won't hurt your chances for funding, either.

Third, on a few rare occasions, it may be the case that no member of the standing advisory subcommittee is expert in the content area of a specific proposal. Let me quickly emphasize that this is indeed rare: panel members are chosen to represent many areas of the field, and generally have broad knowledge outside their own specialties. But four persons cannot possibly represent *every* interest or line of research in a field as diverse as social psychology. (Remember: at NSF two of the six members of the panel are developmental psychologists.) For this reason, it may well be worth your while to obtain the names of current members of the advisory panel. (This information is available upon request.) If, after learning the identity of these persons, you feel that none has sufficient expertise in the area of your proposal, discuss this matter with the Program Director. Several steps are open in such cases (e.g., the Program Director may decide to seek a larger number of ad hoc reviews than is usual; she or he may seek input from scientists working at the foundation, or those on other advisory panels.) But these steps may not be instituted unless you call the situation to the program officer's attention early in the game. Thus, once again, my advice is simple: when in doubt, communicate with the appropriate person. Your concern and input will be appreciated, and may well serve to improve the overall quality of the review process with respect to your proposal.

A note on chance: Is peer review really "random"? During my tenure at NSF, I often heard the following remark from colleagues (in many cases, from ones whose proposals had recently been declined): "Oh well, it's all a matter of luck anyway." What they meant by such comments was this: whether a given proposal is supported or declined depends, to an important degree, on the "luck of the draw"—who, specifically, happens to review it. Implicit in this suggestion is the belief that there is little consensus among one's colleagues with respect to the merits of various proposals. Presented with the same document, some will rate it highly, others will view it as mediocre, and still others will rate it as totally inadequate. To the extent this is so, the fate of a specific proposal will, in fact, depend on who happens to receive it. Is there any validity to this contention? Unfortunately, a study by Cole, Cole, and Simon (1981) suggests that there is. These investigators had 150 proposals, previously submitted to NSF and evaluated by its expert consultants, evaluated once again by a second independent set of reviewers. (The proposals were in the fields of chemistry, economics, and physics—not psychology.) Results were far from comforting. In general, there was little agreement between the ratings provided by the two sets of reviewers. Indeed, the level of disagreement was such that the following conclusion was supported: whether a given proposal would be funded depended very strongly on which persons happened to review it.

In a sense, these results, disturbing as they are, are hardly surprising. In the final analysis, each proposal must be evaluated by specific persons. Given the complexity of the task they face, and differences in their background, perspective, and subjective weightings for various features of proposals, contrasting ratings are only to be expected. Indeed, it would be much more surprising if the judgments of individual reviewers always coincided. The fact that such differences exist, however, does *not* imply that the judgmental process is totally random—far from it. While disagreements do exist, I was struck, while at NSF, by the large number of proposals about which there was a high degree of consensus in reviewer sentiment. Further, there is an important safeguard built into the system, and designed to reduce the impact of the type of chance factors mentioned above. Specifically, this involves the fact that panel members examine all reviews of each proposal, as well as the proposal itself. An important part of their task at panel meetings, then, is that of considering disparate evaluations, and determining which ones should carry maximum weight. This procedure, I believe, goes a long way toward reducing the possibility that "bad luck" in the assignment of external reviewers, or in the pattern of which individuals actually return written reviews, will doom a proposal to failure. Of course, this is not to say that the impact of such chance factors is totally eliminated in this manner. Who reads a given proposal *does* sometimes make a difference. Thus, while every effort is made to hold the impact of this variable to a minimum, it does represent an important way in which "noise" can enter the review process.

To conclude: the peer review system—good as it usually is—does leave room for certain sources of error. You should be aware of this fact, and do everything in your power to help the program director and panel in their efforts to minimize such difficulties. To the extent you do, you will contribute to the fairness and informativeness of the review process. And maximizing these attributes is a central goal of the entire system.

SUBMITTING A RESEARCH PROPOSAL: WHO, WHAT, HOW AND HOW MUCH?

It is often said that there is a "right" and a "wrong" way to do just about everything. While the accuracy of this statement can probably be questioned in certain spheres of life (ones where personal taste is of central importance), there is little doubt that it does apply to submitting research proposals. Countless times during my two years at NSF I fervently wished that someone would do *something* about getting this point across to my colleagues. Indeed, my recollections of these many painful instances constitute one of my prime motives for preparing this chapter. And while I'm not usually given to excessive bursts of euphoria, I am somewhat hopeful that the following information will help save principal investigators much time, effort, and energy in the years ahead.

Who: Where to Submit a Specific Proposal

After months of hard work—and with a dollop of inspiration—you've developed what you feel is a truly excellent program of research. In fact, you are sure that it's nothing short of spectacular—a major breakthrough if ever there was one. You can't wait to get it into the mail. But now, you face a very practical decision: to which agency (or agencies) do you send it? After examining some 400 separate proposals at NSF, it's my considered opinion that many of my colleagues proceed under the following general guideline: "Who cares—the more the better!" In one sense, of course, this is reasonable. In these days of tight (one might almost say "vanishing") budgets, it does make sense to submit a given proposal to as many potential sources as possible. But in another, it makes little sense indeed.

Specific federal agencies—and often, specific units within them—have restrictions on the type of research they can fund. At NSF, for example, there is a general policy that forbids the funding of clinical research. The precise meaning of "clinical" varies over time, but as you might guess, it tends to become somewhat broader at times when budgets are on the wane. Similarly, during the period I worked at NSF, there was a firm policy prohibiting the funding of applied research in the basic research programs. Again, there is certainly room for maneuver or discussion with respect to the precise meaning of "applied." But this policy, too, was real, and often strictly enforced.

What happens, then, when a heedless principal investigator submits a proposal lying outside the jurisdiction of a particular funding agency, or one that is expressly eliminated from consideration by firm policy? Unfortunately, nothing good. The proposal, of course, *cannot* be funded. Indeed, often it cannot even be reviewed. But it does add to the work-load of all persons concerned, and can contribute to the clogging of important channels of communication. Further, the receipt of a proposal at one agency may delay its processing at another, and more appropriate, agency. (The same research cannot be funded by two agencies at once; thus, when a proposal has been sent to several different units, the program officers involved must coordinate their actions. And this can require precious time.) Finally, investigators should not overlook the negative affect that may be generated among program officers and other persons who must deal with the proposal—negative affect that may become associated with the investigator and persist far longer than he or she might wish.

By now, I trust, the message I am trying to communicate is clear. Put very simply it is "*Look before you leap*." Before sending multiple copies of a multiple-page proposal, check with the person on the receiving end to be certain that it is going to an appropriate destination. A few phone calls at this stage of the process can save you—and many other persons—a great deal of pointless effort.

What: The Content of Research Proposals

Inspiration, in science as in other creative fields, is a personal thing. Thus, the precise contents of a research proposal must derive from each investigator's unique blend of knowledge, intuition, and insight. Any attempt to specify the form or nature of this process here would be both pointless and presumptuous. Yet, at the same time, there *are* some general considerations concerning the scope of proposals and how they should be prepared that may be worth noting. Some of these are now outlined.

Let's begin at the beginning: how, precisely, do you start? One useful answer, especially for young investigators, is this: obtain copies of successful proposals submitted by your colleagues. In short, examine several proposals that have already been funded. Studying these will often yield useful ideas about the overall organization, length, and scope of your own proposal. Further, it may help you avoid several pitfalls that lie in wait for unwary novices. For these reasons, the value of beginning with an in-depth study of several models of what a good proposal should be like cannot be overstated.

Next, let's consider the question of detail. How much is enough? This issue arises most frequently with respect to specific procedures to be followed in a research program. Most investigators are well aware of the appropriate level of detail where journal articles are concerned. For some reason, though, they seem to lose sight of such guidelines when preparing research proposals. As a result, reviewers often complain either that they do not have enough information at their disposal to fully evaluate this aspect of a project, or that they have too much—that they are literally drowning in unnecessary specifics. Both of these outcomes are clearly to be avoided. The basic guideline to follow, therefore, is this: provide reviewers of the propsal with enough information to form a clear picture of just what will be done—how, precisely, the proposed studies will be conducted. At the same time, though, avoid loading them down with so many details that they soon forget just why the project is important and what, in terms of major goals, it seeks to accomplish.

Finally, a word on the value of *pre-submission* feedback. After you've prepared your proposal, *do not* simply go ahead and submit it. Instead, seek the comments and evaluations of several of your colleagues before sending it to the appropriate agencies. The feedback they provide can prove invaluable in calling attention to potential difficulties in planned procedures, points of weakness in your theory, and other matters. If you don't obtain this feedback before submitting the proposal, chances are good that you will receive it later—as part of your official notification that it has been declined!

How: Why Rules—Silly as They May Seem—Really Count

At many universities, the statement "Rules are made to be broken" is at least partially true. Where the federal government is concerned, however, it rarely applies. Thus, when you prepare a research proposal for submission to a federal granting agency, it is *absolutely, positively, unconditionally* essential that you pay attention to the mechanics of the process. That is, you must devote careful attention to following the rules for submission established by the particular agency or agencies with which you wish to deal. To make life more complicated, each agency often insists on slightly different things. But all have *some* guidelines on how proposals are to be typed, their length, dates of submission, and so on. These rules may strike you as silly and excessively bureaucratic; and you are right—they are. But still, they *must* be followed. The consequences of failing to do so can be costly indeed.

For example, the unit of NSF where I worked (the Division of Behavioral and Neural Sciences) had a standing rule that the body of all research proposals (the portion that actually describes the research planned, etc.) could not be more than 19 pages in length. Departures from this basic guideline were permitted only in rare cases, and with prior consent of the appropriate Program Director. Imagine my chagrin, then, when each month I received several proposals 30, 40, 50, or more pages in length! I then faced the highly unpleasant task of phoning these colleagues, and informing them that their gargantuan labors had been in vain: I could not even send their proposal out for review until it had been reduced to the required number of pages. Clearly, this often presented such persons with major difficulties; indeed, I'm afraid that there may still be one or two individuals who will avoid me at conventions in the years ahead, because of their firm belief that somehow, I was directly responsible for their suffering. Actually, of course, it stemmed from a far less personal basis: their failure to check before proceeding.

Another point worth considering when you prepare a proposal involves deadlines for submission. I would estimate that fully half of all the proposals I received during my stay at NSF arrived with no prior communication from the principal investigator. True, NSF does not have firm deadlines for receipt of proposals—they can be submitted and received at any time. But from a practical point of view, work must still be batched. Obviously, if panel members are to read through 50–60 proposals, they must receive these all at once—not in dribs and drabs. Similarly, when proposals are sent out to ad hoc consultants, sufficient time must be provided for these documents to reach the reviewers, be examined, and returned to the foundation prior to the next scheduled panel meeting. For these and other reasons (e.g., efficient use of the semi-automated mailing system), only proposals received by a specific date can be reviewed at a given panel meeting. Despite the reasonable nature of these considerations, though, many principal investigators—including experienced ones—never bothered to check with me about such dates. As a result, they were much chagrined to learn that their proposals had arrived too late to be included in the next panel meeting. Finally, a similar situation existed with respect to starting dates. NSF (and all other federal agencies) are large and somewhat bureaucratic organizations. Thus, even after a proposal is reviewed and recommended for support by a Program Director, it must pass through many steps before an actual grant is made. For example, it must be examined and approved by the Division Director, it must be certified by the Division of Finance and Accounting, and finally, it must be closely examined by the Division of Grants and Contracts. All of this takes time—usually, a bare minimum of 6–7 months from the time a proposal is received until the award of a formal grant. This information is published in several NSF documents, and is included in information produced by each Program and available on request. Yet, I regularly received proposals with starting dates only three, two, or even one month away. (In fact, I received a few proposals that arrived *after* their proposed start date: talk about optimism!!) In a more serious vein, some of these documents contained information in their budgets suggesting that firm commitments had been made to individuals and businesses on the basis of these unrealistic start dates. Clearly, major problems could well arise in such cases. And again, all these problems might easily have been avoided if the investigators in question had followed my simple rule: when in doubt (and even if *not* in doubt), check ahead; the misery you save may be your own!

By the way, I should note that University Grants Offices are often *not* the best sources of information on such matters. Rules and guidelines change fairly often, and frequently, Grants Offices are not very up-to-date in this respect. Even worse, I encountered many cases in which they had actually given false and misleading information about deadlines, length, and so on to my colleagues. For these reasons, then, I strongly recommend that you get your information directly from the source—right from the agency or program to which you wish to apply for research support.

In any case, when submitting a proposal, please, *please,* **PLEASE** do pay careful attention to the mechanical details. Find out how it should be typed and prepared, how many copies should be sent, to whom they should be mailed, and by what date. Failing to do so may well yield a bitter harvest of delay, extra work, and shattered dreams.

How Much? Where Budgets Are Concerned, Don't Let Your Ego Be Your Guide

People often have many different reasons for doing the things they do. In other words, much of human behavior stems from a complex array of multiple motives. And my experience at NSF suggests that writing and submitting research proposals, too, can be described in these terms. Persons submitting such proposals (including, of course, myself!) seem to have the following concurrent motives: (1) obtaining financial support for a research project that could not be conducted (or conducted as well) in the absence of these funds; (2) gaining the prestige and status that go along with such awards; (3) yielding to external pressures from their department or University which suggest that submitting proposals is definitely "the thing to do"; and (4) aggrandizing their ego or self-image. In general, these motives are of no particular interest to the peer review system. Its job is simply that of evaluating the quality and value of the planned research. The motives behind any given project are largely irrelevant. But there is one place in all proposals where the precise "mix" of these motives often becomes vividly and sometimes painfully apparent: the budget.

During my two years at NSF, I examined several hundred proposals and their accompanying budget. My overall conclusion: social psychologists differ tremendously in terms of the motives behind their proposal-writing activities. Many (most, I believe) seem genuinely concerned with obtaining financial support so that they may conduct valuable research. Thus, the sums requested in their budgets are both moderate and reasonable. But others, I'm afraid, seem more concerned with points (2) and (4) above. Their budgets often represent exercises in what might be termed *empire founding* or *ego-aggrandizement.* In more concrete terms, the budgets I examined during my stay at NSF ranged from modest (perhaps overly modest) requests for only $10,000-15,000 during an 18-month period, through a request for $1.4 million for a 5-year period! Fortunately, the great majority of the budgets I saw were reasonable—they requested levels of support that with today's large overhead would yield only enough funds for modest equipment purchases, the services of one or two half-time assistants, and perhaps a part-time secretary or technician. (The figure required for such support currently seems to be about $50,000 in total funding—i.e., direct and indirect costs—per year.) But I also vividly recall dozens of projects that requested two, three, or even five times this level of support. Needless to add, some research projects *are* more expensive to conduct than others. Yet, this factor did not seem to be the major one underlying these huge differences in levels of requested funding. Indeed, projects involving comparable methods of data collection and analysis, and requiring the services of similar numbers of staff, would often vary by a factor of two or three with respect to total budgets. Thus, I (and other persons involved in the review process) could only conclude that factors unrelated to the actual conduction of the research were at work.

But what are the effects of budgets on the fate of various proposals? Ostensibly, there should be none. NSF and other granting agencies have as policy this idea: the scientific merit of a proposal should be assessed separately and distinctly from the level of support it requests. As social psychologists, though, we realize that this is not totally feasible. How, after all, can reviewers of a given project fail to take account of the budget? Most are active, experienced researchers, who have a good idea of the level of support actually needed for the conduction of a specific series of studies. Thus, it is far from surprising that often they become quite irritated or annoyed with budgets that request several times the amount of support they deem to be appropriate. And once such anger is evoked, it can readily color perceptions and evaluations of an entire project, despite the best efforts of the persons involved to avoid such effects. Clearly, this is an outcome most investigators will definitely wish to avoid.

In their own defense, individuals who submit large and inflated budgets often argue that they *must* follow this strategy, since their requests are certain to be deeply slashed. While this argument seems compelling, I can assure you that it is largely spurious in nature. The guiding rule at NSF and other funding agencies is simple: provide investigators with the levels of support they actually need to successfully conduct their projects. There are *no* fixed rules concerning budget reductions, and certainly no requirement that all budgets be reduced by a fixed percentage. Thus, during my tenure as a Program Director, I recomended funding at precisely the levels requested in many proposals: the budget for these projects were eminently reasonable, so there were no grounds for reducing them whatsoever. In cases where budgets *were* excessive, though, reductions of up to 60%–70% were made.

Incidentally, it is usually wise to discuss your budget with the chair of your department before submitting a proposal. Each department has its own guidelines concerning priorities and level of funding for graduate students, secretaries, computer time, work by the departmental shop, and so on. Details concerning each of these items should be arranged in advance so that misunderstandings can be avoided. Similarly, any special needs connected with the research (e.g., the need for increased laboratory space, structural modifications) should also be considered prior to submission. If they are left until after a proposal has been funded, the start of the project—or even its ultimate feasibility—may be placed in jeopardy.

In sum, when you prepare the budget to accompany a research proposal, my advice is as follows: *request only the level of support you really need.* And if you err, it is probably to do so on the side of being too modest. Allowing your budget to become an exercise in self-aggrandizement or empire building may improve your mood and enhance your ego, but in the end, it may prove *very* costly. Thus, I urge you to avoid it in all cases.

The "Seven Deadly Sins" of Proposal Writing: Common Pitfalls to Avoid

Even when times were relatively "good" for psychology (note the quotation marks around "good"!), research grants were a scarce commodity. As I noted earlier, miniscule budgets assured that no more than 20% of the proposals received could be funded; and this figure was often substantially lower. Attaining federal support, then, has always been a highly competitive undertaking. Are there any techniques for gaining an "edge" in this contest—tactics for enhancing your chances of success? Actually, I believe that there are. While I certainly can't offer you a magic formula for submitting "no-fail" proposals, I *can* at least warn you against a number of common pitfalls—snares that often derail promising ideas and projects very early in the game. My comments in this regard stem mainly from my experience at NSF, where I was exposed to written and verbal comments about hundreds of separate proposals. But they also derive from conversations with my counterparts at other granting agencies. Thus, I believe that they are fairly general in scope.

"Sin" #1: The Absence of Theory: Perhaps the most common flaw in the proposals whose evaluation I witnessed was the lack of a clearly stated theory. Many otherwise promising proposals—ones that focused

on intriguing research questions and offered ingenious approaches to them—went down to quick defeat simply because they contained no unifying theoretical framework. Please note: such frameworks do *not* have to be extensive or fully developed; after all, their refinement is often one major goal sought in the overall project. But *some* underlying theory should be presented. In the total absence of such conceptualization, the chances for funding are quite remote.

"Sin" #2: The Absence of Clear-cut Links Between Theory and Research: A related issue involves the existence (and explication) of clear conceptual links between the theory proposed, and the research studies planned. Unfortunately, all too many proposals fall into the following "trap": they offer an intriguing theory, and describe interesting and carefully planned studies. But then, they omit clear conceptual links between these two basic components. In short, the theory presented does not appear to "drive" the studies and any results obtained will not be useful in assessing the theory's adequacy. This is an important potential weakness, and one worth considering with care before you submit any proposal.

"Sin" #3: Methodological Flaws or Ambiguity: Many additional proposals are downrated either because they contain obvious flaws in methodology, or simply because of ambiguity in this respect. In the former case, interpretation of the obtained results is problematic, and the overall value of the project is sharply reduced. In the latter instance, assessments of the adequacy of the proposed methods cannot be made: there is simply not enough evidence for making such judgments. In both cases, decline of the proposal is almost certain. Before submitting, therefore, you should give careful attention to both issues. First, be sure that your methodology is sound. And second, be certain that it is described in sufficient detail for persons not intimately familiar with it to grasp its major points. In both of these respects, the opinions and advice of colleagues can prove invaluable. Thus, it is always useful to seek their input on these issues before proceeding.

"Sin" #4: The Absence of Close Links to Past, Related Work: In my experience, many otherwise excellent proposals are downrated for a simple and easily avoided reason: they fail to take adequate account of past work on the same or related topics. Recall that panel members and ad hoc consultants are often experts in the topics examined by a given proposal. Thus, they object very strongly when they note that a principal investigator seems to be working in something akin to a "conceptual vacuum." Always be careful, therefore, to point out links between your own proposed research and similar work in the extant literature. If you do not, someone else is bound to do so—often in a highly critical manner.

"Sin" #5: An Absence of Overall Significance for the Field: While the

technical factors considered above are all crucial, they are not the only points considered when a proposal is evaluated. In addition, panel members and ad hoc consultants also frequently take a step back from these matters, and address a more general issue: will the findings of the project—even if uniformly positive—offer a substantial contribution to the field? In short, will they contribute in measurable ways to the growth and development of social psychology? The reason for asking this question is clear: reviewers generally know that funds are so limited that not even all theoretically and technically sound proposals can be supported. Thus, they recognize that the border issue of relative contribution to the field, too, must be considered. Before you submit, therefore, you should also take a step back from your work and cast a jaundiced eye over its potential benefits for social psychology. And if these are not obvious, give some thought to the task of making them so.

"Sin" #6: Inappropriate or Ambiguous Plans for Data Analysis: Often, investigators seem to devote surprisingly little attention to a key question relating to their research: how will the data collected be analyzed or reduced? Both panel members and ad hoc consultants frequently comment on this issue. Thus, when clear and appropriate plans for data analysis are not presented, they often sharply downrate otherwise impressive proposals. For this reason, you should take pains to specify your major plans in this respect with care. (Please note: great detail is *not* needed. But some concrete plan for data reduction should be included.)

"Sin" #7: Proposing Too Much or Proposing Too Little: A final common pitfall into which many proposals seem to tumble is quite prosaic: proposing to do too much, or proposing to do too little. Again, keep in mind the fact that reviewers of all proposals are generally experienced researchers themselves. Thus, they have a good "feel" for how much work can be accomplished in a given time period, within a specific area of investigation. It is important, therefore, that you give careful thought to this issue before submitting. Erring seriously in either direction can be costly in terms of overall reviewer assessments.

The "seven deadly sins": A concluding comment. At this point, I should hasten to note that even taking careful account of all the potential problems listed above cannot, of course, guarantee success. Many other factors enter into the evaluation of specific research projects, and these are too numerous to consider here. In my opinion, though, the weaknesses just noted are among the most serious and among the most common. Indeed, they often serve to remove even promising proposals from further consideration as soon as they are identified. Thus, if you manage to avoid them, you will be off to a strong start. At the least, you will probably avoid that first, deadly "cut," and this in itself is a major positive accomplishment.

AND THEN WHAT? OBLIGATIONS AFTER RECEIVING A GRANT

Imagine that, to paraphrase Voltaire, it is the best of all possible worlds, at least where your research is concerned. You have just been notified that your grant proposal has been approved and will definitely be funded. Is that the end of our story? Do you now simply go off on your merry way, performing the research you planned, and following up interesting leads as they arise? In fact, many investigators seem to adopt just this strategy. Once their proposal is funded, all communication from them ceases (except perhaps, for the required, brief progress reports). And it only resumes as the time for renewal or reapplication rolls around once again.

Such reactions are perfectly understandable. We are all wrapped up in our work, and tend to concentrate on it to the exclusion of many other things. But when principal investigators "take the money and run," so to speak, they miss out on an important opportunity to aid their field. Let me clarify why this is so.

During my time at NSF, I was repeatedly called upon to prepare reports designed to illustrate the value and appeal of social psychology. Some of these took the form of one-page "nuggets"—brief descriptions of specific projects or intriguing, recent findings that could be turned into press releases by the Foundation's Office of Information. Others were longer documents—for example, commentary on the outlook for further progress in the field during the years ahead. And on several occasions, I was asked to deliver brief verbal presentations to high-ranking officers of the Foundation, and to members of the National Science Board. These, too, were designed to emphasize the strength and value of our field. In most of these instances, the content of my written or verbal reports was not specified in any manner. Indeed, the only restriction was that my comments be based upon research projects currently funded by NSF. With this requirement in mind, I naturally drew heavily on the progress reports, reprints, and preprints sent to me by principal investigators. Thus, in a crucial sense, the quality and up-to-dateness of my reports rested heavily on this vital input. The better and more complete it was, the more effective I could be in representing social psychology at NSF, and in Washington.

For this reason, it is important that principal investigators remain in close touch with the agencies supporting their research throughout the tenure of their grants. In particular, they should spare no effort in keeping the Program Director or other administrative official fully informed of their progress. And they should take special pains to call any new and exciting findings to her or his attention at once. Doing so arms this person with ammunition that may prove vital in the continuing struggle to convince society as a whole, and Congress in particular, of the value of committing limited resources to the support of such work. Of course, even this information, coupled with the very best efforts of spokespersons for our field, cannot guarantee a positive outcome. The unsettling events of 1981 brought this point sharply into focus—and with a vengeance. Yet, they are certainly steps in the right direction. And at this point in time, with strong political currents running against us, they are probably needed more than ever.

One final point: once you have been funded, is it necessary to stick strictly to the plan you initially proposed? That is, must you perform all of the studies you outlined, and only those studies? The answer is an emphatic No! NSF and other funding agencies permit a considerable degree of flexibility. If investigators uncover unexpected findings, or encounter unpredicted phenomena, they are encouraged to shift gears and actively pursue these new leads. All that is required is that they discuss alterations in their research plans with appropriate officials, and then keep them informed of subsequent progress. The ultimate goal, after all, is a contribution to scientific knowledge, *not* the completion of some rigid plan or time-table.

To conclude: principal investigators should not view the receipt of a research grant as the end of the process. Rather, they should perceive it as the start of a significant working relationship between themselves and the funding agency—one in which the support they receive obligates them to report fully and promptly on their work. Clearly, this can be a chore—one more item to add to our busy schedules. But given the potential benefits that can result from such close cooperation, I firmly believe it is a task investigators should be more than willing to perform. And please keep one final point in mind: in the nation's capital—as in more saintly provinces—the greatest amount of help usually goes to those (those fields or professions) who do the most on their own behalf!

REFERENCE

Cole, S., Cole, J. R., & Simon, G. A. (1981). Chance and consensus in peer review. *Science, 214,* 881–886.

8
WRITING THE EMPIRICAL JOURNAL ARTICLE

Daryl J. Bem
Cornell University

You have conducted a study and analyzed the data. Now it is time to write. To publish. To tell the world what you have learned. The purpose of this chapter is to enhance the chances that some journal editor will let you do so.

If you are new to this enterprise, you may find it helpful to consult two additional sources of information. For detailed information on the proper format of a journal article, see the *Publication Manual of the American Psychological Association* (APA, 1983) and recent articles in the journal to which you plan to submit your manuscript. For renewing your acquaintance with the formal and stylistic elements of English prose, you can read Chapter 2 of the *Publication Manual* or any one of several style manuals. I recommend *The Elements of Style* by Strunk and White (1979). It is brief, witty, and inexpensive.

Because I write, review, and edit primarily for journals in personality and social psychology, I have drawn most of my examples from those areas. Colleagues assure me, however, that the guidelines set forth here are also pertinent for articles in experimental psychology and biopsychology. Similarly, this chapter focuses on the report of an empirical study, but the general writing suggestions apply as well to the theoretical articles, literature reviews, and methodological contributions that also appear in our journals.

PLANNING IT

Which Article Should You Write?

There are two possible articles you can write: (1) the article you planned to write when you designed your study or (2) the article that makes the most sense now that you have seen the results. They are rarely the same, and the correct answer is (2).

The conventional view of the research process is that we first derive a set of hypotheses from a theory, design and conduct a study to test these hypotheses, analyze the data to see if they were confirmed or disconfirmed, and then chronicle this sequence of events in the journal article. If this is how our enterprise actually proceeded, we could write most of the article before we collected the data. We could write the introduction and method sections completely, prepare the results section in skeleton form, leaving spaces to be filled in by the specific numerical results, and have two possible discussion sections ready to go, one for positive results, the other for negative results.

But this is not how our enterprise actually proceeds. Psychology is more exciting than that, and the best journal articles are informed by the actual empirical findings from the opening sentence. Before writing your article, then, you need to Analyze Your Data. Herewith, a sermonette on the topic.

Analyzing Data. Once upon a time, psychologists observed behavior directly, often for sustained periods of time. No longer. Now, the higher the investigator goes up the tenure ladder, the more remote he or she typically becomes from the grounding observations of our science. If you are already a successful research psychologist, then you probably haven't seen a subject for some time. Your graduate assistant assigns the running of a study to a bright undergraduate who writes the computer program that collects the data automatically. And like the modern dentist, the modern psychologist rarely even sees the data until they have been cleaned by human or computer hygienists.

To compensate for this remoteness from our subjects, let us at least become intimately familiar with the record of their behavior: the data. Examine them from every angle. Analyze the sexes separately. Make up new composite indices. If a datum suggests a new hypothesis, try to find further evidence for it elsewhere in the data. If you see dim traces of interesting patterns, try to reorganize the data to bring them into bolder relief. If there are subjects you don't like, or trials, observers or interviewers who gave you anomalous results, drop them (temporarily). Go on a fishing expedition for something—anything—interesting.

No, this is not immoral. The rules of scientific and statistical inference that we overlearn in graduate school apply to the "Context of Justification." They tell us what we can conclude in the articles we write for public consumption, and they give our readers criteria for deciding whether or not to believe us. But in the "Context of Discovery," there are no formal rules, only heuristics or strategies. How does one discover a new phenomenon? Smell a good idea? Have a brilliant insight into behavior? Create a new theory? In the confining context of an empirical study, there is only one strategy for discovery: exploring the data.

Yes, there is a danger. Spurious findings can emerge by chance, and we need to be cautious about anything we discover in this way. In limited cases, there are statistical techniques that correct for this danger. But there are no statistical correctives for overlooking an important discovery because we were insufficiently attentive to the data. Let us err on the side of discovery.

Reporting the Findings. When you are through exploring, you may conclude that the data are not strong enough to justify your new insights formally, but at least you are now ready to design the "right" study. If you still plan to report the current data, you may wish to mention the new insights tentatively, stating honestly that they remain to be tested adequately. Alternatively, the data may be strong enough to justify recentering your article around the new findings and subordinating or even ignoring your original hypotheses.

This is not advice to suppress negative results. If your study was genuinely designed to test hypotheses that derive from a formal theory or are of wide general interest for some other reason, then they should remain the focus of your article. The integrity of the scientific enterprise requires the reporting of disconfirming results.

But this requirement assumes that somebody out there cares about the hypotheses. Many respectable studies are explicitly exploratory or are launched from speculations of the "I-wonder-if . . ." variety. If your study is one of these, then nobody cares if you were wrong. Contrary to the conventional wisdom, science does not care how clever or clairvoyant you were at guessing your results ahead of time. Scientific integrity does not require you to lead your readers through all your wrongheaded hunches only to show—*voila!*—they were wrongheaded. A journal article should not be a personal history of your stillborn thoughts.

Your overriding purpose is to tell the world what you have learned from your study. If your results suggest a compelling framework for their presentation, adopt it and make the most instructive findings your centerpiece. Think of your data as a jewel. Your task is to cut and polish it, to select the facets to highlight, and to craft the best setting for it. Many experienced authors write the results section first.

But before writing anything, Analyze Your Data!

End of sermonette.

How Should You Write?

The primary criteria for good scientific writing are accuracy and clarity. If your article is interesting and written with style, fine. But these are subsidiary virtues. First strive for accuracy and clarity.

The first step toward clarity is good organization, and the standardized format of a journal article does much of the work for you. It not only permits readers to read the report from beginning to end, as they would any coherent narrative, but also to scan it for a quick overview of the study or to locate specific information easily by turning directly to the relevant section. Within that format, however, it is still helpful to work from an outline of your own. This enables you to examine the logic of the sequence, to spot important points that are omitted or misplaced, and to decide how best to divide the labor of presentation between the introduction and final discussion (about which, more later).

The second step toward clarity is to write simply and directly. A journal article tells a straightforward tale of a circumscribed problem in search of a solution. It is not a novel with subplots, flashbacks, and literary allusions, but a short story with a single, linear, narrative line. Let this line stand out in bold relief. Don't make your voice struggle to be heard above the ambient noise of cluttered writing. You are justifiably proud of your 90th percentile verbal aptitude, but let it nourish your prose, not glut it. Write simply and directly.

For Whom Should You Write?

Scientific journals are published for specialized audiences who share a common background of substantive knowledge and methodological expertise. If you wish to write well, you should ignore this fact. Psychology encompasses a broader range of subjects and methodologies than do most other disciplines, and its findings are frequently of interest to a wider public. The social psychologist should be able to read a *Psychometrika* article on LISREL; the personality theorist, a biopsychology article on hypothalamic function; and the congressional aide with a BA in history, a *Journal of Personality and Social Psychology* article on attribution theory.

Accordingly, good writing is good teaching. Direct your writing to the student in Psychology 100, your colleague in the Art History Department, and your grandmother. No matter how technical or abstruse your article is in its particulars, intelligent nonpsychologists with no expertise in statistics or experimental design should be able to comprehend the broad outlines of what you did and why. They should understand in general terms what was learned. And above all, they should appreciate why someone—anyone—should give a damn. The introduction and discussion sections in particular should be accessible to this wider audience.

The actual technical materials—those found primarily in the method and results sections—should be aimed at a reader one level of expertise less specialized than the audience for which the journal is primarily published. Assume that the reader of your article in *Psychometrika* knows about regression, but needs some introduction to LISREL. Assume that the reader of the *Journal of Personality and Social Psychology* knows about person perception but needs some introduction to dispositional and situational attributions.

Many of the writing techniques suggested in this chapter are thus teaching techniques designed to make your article comprehensible to the widest possible audience. They are also designed to remain invisible or transparent to your readers, thereby infusing your prose with a "subliminal pedagogy." Good writing is good teaching.

WRITING IT

The Shape of an Article

An article is written in the shape of an hourglass. It begins with broad general statements, progressively narrows down to the specifics of your study, and then broadens out again to more general considerations. Thus:

The introduction begins broadly:	"Individuals differ radically from one another in the degree to which they are willing and able to express their emotions."
It becomes more specific:	"Indeed, the popular view is that such emotional expressiveness is a central difference between men and women. . . . But the research evidence is mixed . . ."
And more so:	"There is even some evidence that men may actually . . ."
Until you are ready to introduce your own study in conceptual terms:	"In this study, we recorded the emotional reactions of both men and women to filmed . . ."
The method and results sections are the most specific, the "neck" of the hourglass:	"(Method) One hundred male and 100 female undergraduates were shown one of two movies . . ." "(Results) Table 1 shows that men in the father-watching condition cried significantly more . . ."
The discussion section begins with the implications of your study:	"These results imply that sex differences in emotional expressiveness are moderated by two kinds of variables . . ."

It becomes broader:	"Not since Charles Darwin's first observations has psychology contributed as much new . . ."
And more so:	"If emotions can incarcerate us by hiding our complexity, at least their expression can liberate us by displaying our authenticity."

This closing statement might be a bit grandiose for some journals—I'm not even sure what it means—but if your study is carefully executed and conservatively interpreted, most editors will permit you to indulge yourself a bit at the two broad ends of the hourglass. Being dull only appears to be a prerequisite for publishing in the professional journals.

The Introduction

The Opening Statements. The first task of the article is to introduce the background and nature of the problem being investigated. Here are four rules of thumb for your opening statements:

1. Write in English prose, not psychological jargon.
2. Don't plunge unprepared readers into the middle of your problem or theory. Take the time and space necessary to lead them up to the formal or theoretical statement of the problem step by step.
3. Use examples to illustrate theoretical points or to introduce unfamiliar conceptual or technical terms. The more abstract the material, the more important such examples become.
4. Whenever possible, try to open with a statement about people (or animals), not psychologists or their research. (This rule is almost always violated. Don't use journals as a model here.)

Examples of Opening Statements:

Wrong: Recently, Ekman (1972), Izard (1977), Tomkins (1980), and Zajonc (1980) have pointed to psychology's neglect of the affects and their expression. [Okay for somewhere in the introduction, but not the opening statement.]

Right: Individuals differ radically from one another in the degree to which they are willing and able to express their emotions.

Wrong: Research in the forced-compliance paradigm has focused on the effects of predecisional alternatives and incentive magnitude.

Wrong: Festinger's theory of cognitive dissonance has received a great deal of attention during the past 20 years.

> *Right:* The individual who holds two beliefs that are inconsistent with one another may feel uncomfortable. For example, the person who knows that he or she enjoys smoking but believes it to be unhealthy may experience discomfort arising from the inconsistency or disharmony between these two thoughts or cognitions. This feeling of discomfort has been called *cognitive dissonance* by social psychologist Leon Festinger (1957), who suggests that individuals will be motivated to remove this dissonance in whatever way they can.

Note how this last example leads the reader from familiar terms (beliefs, inconsistency, discomfort, thoughts) through transition terms (disharmony, cognitions) to the unfamiliar technical terms *cognitive dissonance,* thereby providing an explicit, if nontechnical, definition of it. The following example illustrates how one might define a technical term (ego control) and identify its conceptual status (a personality variable) more implicitly:

> The need to delay gratification, control impulses, and modulate emotional expression is the earliest and most ubiquitous demand that society places upon the developing child. And because success at so many of life's tasks depends critically upon the individual's mastery of such ego control, evidence for life-course continuities in this central personality domain should be readily obtained.

And finally, here is an example in which the technical terms are defined only by the context. Note, however, that the technical abbreviation, MAO, is still identified explicitly when it is first introduced.

> In the continuing search for the biological correlates of psychiatric disorder, blood platelets are now a prime target of investigation. In particular, reduced monoamine oxidase (MAO) activity in the platelets is sometimes correlated with paranoid symptomatology, auditory hallucinations or delusions in chronic schizophrenia, and a tendency towards psychopathology in normal men. Unfortunately, these observations have not always replicated, casting doubt on the hypothesis that MAO activity is, in fact, a biological marker in psychiatric disorder. Even the general utility of the platelet model as a key to central nervous system abnormalities in schizophrenia remains controversial. The present study attempts to clarify the relation of MAO activity to symptomatology in chronic schizophrenia.

This kind of writing would not appear in *Newsweek,* and yet it is still comprehensible to an intelligent layperson who may know nothing about blood platelets, MAO activity, or biological markers. The structure of the writing itself adequately defines the relationships among these things and provides enough context to make the basic idea of the study and its rationale clear. At the same time, this introduction is not condescending nor will it bore the technically sophisticated reader. The pedagogy that makes this introduction accessible to the nonspecialist will not only be transparent to the specialist, but will enhance the clarity of the article for both readers.

Examples of Examples. When developing complex conceptual arguments or introducing technical materials, it is important not only to provide your readers with illustrative examples, but to select the examples with care. In particular, you should try to compose one or two examples that anticipate your actual findings and then use them recurrently to make several interrelated conceptual points. For example, in one of my own studies of trait consistency, some subjects were consistently friendly but not consistently conscientious (Bem & Allen, 1974). Accordingly, we used examples of friendliness and conscientiousness throughout the introduction to clarify and illustrate our theoretical points about the subtleties of trait consistency. This pedagogical technique strengthens the thematic coherence of an article and silently prepares the reader for understanding the results. It also shortens the article by removing the need to explain the theory once in the introduction with hypothetical examples and then again in the context of the actual results.

This chapter you are now reading itself provides examples of recurring examples. Although you don't know it yet, the major example will be the fictitious study of sex differences in emotional expression introduced earlier to illustrate the hourglass shape of an article. I deliberately constructed the study and provided a sufficient overview of it at the beginning so that I could draw upon it throughout the chapter. Watch for its elaboration as we proceed. I chose dissonance theory as a second example because most psychologists are already familiar with it; I can draw upon this shared resource without having to expend a lot of space explaining it. But just in case you weren't familiar with it, I introduced it first in the context of "examples of opening statements" where I could bring you in from the beginning—just as you should do with your own readers. And finally, the Bem-Allen article on trait consistency, mentioned in the paragraph above, has some special attributes that will earn it additional cameo appearances as we continue.

The Literature Review. After making the opening statements, summarize the current state of knowledge in the area of investigation. What previous research has been done on the problem? What are the pertinent theories of the phenomenon? Although you will have familiarized yourself with the literature before you designed your own study, you may need to look up additional references if your results raise a new aspect of the problem or lead you to recast the study in a different framework. For example, if you discover an unanticipated sex difference in your data, you will want to determine if others have reported a similar sex difference or findings that might explain it. If you consider this finding important, discuss sex differences and the pertinent literature in the introduction. If you consider it to be only a peripheral finding, then postpone a discussion of sex differences until the discussion section.

The *Publication Manual* gives the following guidelines for the literature review:

> Discuss the literature but do not include an exhaustive historical review. . . . Although you should acknowledge the contributions of others to the study of the problem, cite only that research pertinent to the specific issue and avoid references with only tangential or general significance. If you summarize earlier works, avoid nonessential details; instead, emphasize pertinent findings, relevant methodological issues, and major conclusions. Refer the reader to general surveys or reviews of the topic if they are available. (APA, 1983, p. 25)

The *Publication Manual* also urges authors not to let the goal of brevity mislead them into writing a statement intelligible only to the specialist. One technique for describing even an entire study succinctly without sacrificing clarity is to describe one variation of the procedure in chronological sequence, letting it convey the overview of the study at the same time. (You can use the same technique in your own method section.) Here, for example, is a description of a complicated but classic experiment on cognitive dissonance theory (Festinger & Carlsmith, 1959):

> Sixty male undergraduates were randomly assigned to one of three conditions. In the $1 condition, the subject was first required to perform long repetitive laboratory tasks in an individual experimental session. He was then hired by the experimenter as an "assistant" and paid $1 to tell a waiting fellow student (a confederate) that the tasks were fun and interesting. In the $20 condition, each subject was hired for $20 to do the same thing. In the Control condition, subjects simply engaged in the tasks. After the experiment, each subject indicated on a questionnaire how much he had enjoyed the tasks. The results showed that $1 subjects rated the tasks as significantly more enjoyable than did the $20 subjects, who, in turn, did not differ from the control subjects.

This kind of condensed writing looks easy. It is not, and you will have to rewrite such summaries repeatedly before they are both clear and succinct. The preceding paragraph was the eighth draft.

Citations. The standard journal format permits you to cite authors in the text either by enclosing their last names and the year of publication in parentheses, as in A below, or by using their names in the sentence itself, as in B.

A. "MAO activity in some schizophrenics is actually higher than normal (Tse & Tung, 1949)."
B. "Tse and Tung (1949) report that MAO activity in some schizophrenics is actually higher than normal."

In general, you should use form A, consigning your colleagues to parentheses. Your narrative line should be about MAO activity in schizophrenics, not about Tse and Tung. Occasionally, however, you might want the focus specifically on the authors or researchers: "Theophrastus (280 B.C.) implies that persons are consistent across situations, but Montaigne (1580) insists that they are not. Only Mischel (1968), Peterson (1968), and Vernon (1964), however, have actually surveyed the evidence in detail." The point here is that you have a deliberate choice to make. Don't just intermix the two formats randomly, paying no attention to the narrative structure.

Ending the Introduction. End the introduction with a brief overview of your own study. This provides a smooth transition into the method section, which follows immediately:

> Because this sex difference remains elusive, it seemed desirable to test Zanna's parental-role theory of emotional expression in a more realistic setting. Accordingly, in the study to be presented here, we exposed men and women to filmed scenes designed to evoke either negative or positive emotions and assessed their emotional reactions when they thought they were being observed by one or both of their parents. We also sought to examine the relation of emotional expression to self-esteem.

The Method Section

The *Publication Manuel* spells out in detail what needs to be included in the method section of an article. Here are some additional stylistic suggestions.

If you conducted a fairly complex experiment in which there was a sequence of procedures or events, it is helpful to lead the reader through the sequence as if he or she were a subject. First give the usual overview of the study, including the description of subjects, setting, and variables assessed, but then describe the experiment from the subject's vantage point. Provide summaries or excerpts of what was actually said to the subject, including any rationale or "cover story" that was given. Describe the relevant aspects of the room. Show sample items from questionnaires, labels on attitude scales, copies of stimulus materials and/or pictures of apparatus. If you administered a standard personality test or attitude scale, describe its general properties unless it is very familiar (e.g., the MMPI or the F scale). For example: "Subjects then filled out the Marlowe-Crowne Social Desirability Scale, a true-false inventory that measures the degree to which persons describe themselves in socially desirable terms (e.g., 'I have never lied')."

The purpose of all this is to give your readers a feel for what it was like to be a subject. (This is true even if you used non-human subjects. Thus it is more important to describe the schedule of reinforcement and the inner dimensions of the Skinner Box—what the animal actually saw—than its outer dimensions and the voltage of the power supply.) Such information often bears importantly on the interpretation of the behavior observed, and readers should be in a position to arrive at their own judgments about your conclusions.

Name all groups, variables, and operations with easily recognized and remembered labels. Don't use abbreviations (the AMT5% group) or empty labels (Treatment 3). Instead, tell us about the success group and the failure group, the father-watching condition and the mother-watching condition, the teacher sample and the student sample, and so forth. It is also better to label groups or treatments in operational rather than theoretical terms. It is difficult to remember that it was the high-dissonance group that was offered the small incentive and the low-dissonance group that was offered the large incentive. So tell us instead about the $1 group and the $20 group. You can remind us of the theoretical interpretation of these variables later when you discuss the results.

The method and results sections share the responsibility for presenting certain kinds of data that support the reliability and validity of your substantive findings, and you must judge where this information fits most smoothly into the narrative and when the reader can most easily assimilate it. For example, if you constructed a new personality scale, you need to tell us about its internal homogeneity and other psychometric properties. If you employed observers, tell us about interjudge agreement. If you mailed survey questionnaires, give us the return rate and discuss the possibility that non-respondents differed from respondents. If you discarded certain subjects, tell us why and how many and discuss the possibility that this limits or qualifies the conclusions you can draw. In particular, assure us that they were not all concentrated in the same experimental condition. (Subjects discarded during data analysis should be discussed in the results section.)

Discuss subject dropout problems and other difficulties encountered in executing the study only if they might affect the validity or the interpretation of your results. Otherwise spare us your tales of woe. Do tell us that some subjects fled your high-stress treatment before you could assess their GSR, but do not tell us that your dog ate your pigeon and you had to redo the experiment or that you couldn't run subjects Tuesday night because the custodian inadvertently locked the building.

Manipulations and procedures that yielded no useful information should be mentioned if they were administered before you collected your main data; their presence could have affected your findings. Usually it will be sufficient to say that they yielded no information and will not be discussed further. You probably don't need to mention them at all if they were administered after you collected your main data unless you think that other investigators might try to pursue the same fruitless path. Sometimes, however, a "null" result is surprising or of interest in its own right. In this case, it should be treated as a regular datum in your results section.

After presenting the methods you employed in your study, discuss any ethical issues they might raise. If the research design required you to keep subjects uninformed or even misinformed about the procedures, how did you tell them about this afterwards? How did you obtain their prior consent? Were they free to withdraw at any time? Were they subjected to any embarrassment or discomfort? What steps were followed to protect their anonymity? Were you observing people who were unaware of that fact?

If your study raises any of these issues, you should be prepared to justify your procedures. Moreover, you need to assure us that your subjects were treated with dignity and that they left your study with their self-esteem intact and their respect for you and psychology enhanced rather than diminished. If you used non-human subjects—especially dogs, cats, or primates—then you need to address analogous questions about their care and treatment.

End the method section with a brief summary of the procedure and its overall purpose. Your grandmother should be able to skim the method section without reading it; the final paragraph should bring her back "on line."

The Results Section

In short articles or reports of single empirical studies, the results and discussion are often combined. But if you need to integrate several different kinds of results or discuss several general matters, then prepare a separate discussion section. There is, however, no such thing as pure results section without an accompanying narrative. You cannot just throw numbers at readers and expect them to retain them in memory until they reach the discussion. In other words, write the results section in English prose.

Setting the Stage. Before you can present your results, there are two preliminary matters that need to be handled. First, you should present evidence that your study successfully set up the conditions for testing your hypotheses or answering your questions. If your study required you to produce one group of subjects in a happy mood and another in a depressed mood, show us here that mood ratings made by the two groups were significantly different. If you divided your subjects into groups, assure us that these groups did not differ on some unintended variable that might bear upon the interpretation of your results (e.g., social class, intelligence). If your study required you to misinform subjects about the procedures, how do you know that they were not suspicious, that subjects who participated earlier had not informed subjects who participated later, and that your "cover story" produced the state or belief required for the test of your hypotheses?

Here is also where you can put some of the data discussed above in "The Method Section": Reliabilities of testing instruments, judges, and observers; return rates on mail surveys; and subject dropout problems.

Not all of these matters need to be discussed at the beginning of the results section. In addition to data you think fit better in the method section, some of these other matters might better be postponed until the discussion section when you are considering alternative explanations of your results (e.g., the possibility that some subjects become suspicious). Again, the decision of what to include is very much a matter of judgment. It is an important step, but don't overdo it. Get it out of the way as quickly as possible and get on with your story.

The second preliminary matter to deal with is the method of data analysis. First, describe any overall procedures you used to convert your raw observations into analyzable data. How were responses to your mail survey coded for analysis? How were observers' ratings combined? Were all measures first converted to standard scores? Some of these may also fit better into the method section and need not be repeated here. Similarly, data-combining procedures that are highly specific can be postponed. If you combined three measures of anxiety into a single composite score for analysis, tell us about that later when you are about to present the anxiety data.

Next, tell us about the statistical analysis itself. If this is standard, describe it briefly (e.g., "All data were analyzed by two-way analyses of variance with sex of subject and mood induction as the independent variables"). If the analysis is unconventional or makes certain statistical assumptions your data might not satisfy, however, discuss the rationale for it, perhaps citing a reference for readers who wish to check into it further. If your method of analysis is new or likely to be unfamiliar to readers of the journal, you might need to provide a full explanation of it. Sometimes the quantitative treatment of data is a major part of an article's contribution. Variations of multidimensional scaling, causal modeling, and circumplex representations of personality data, for example, have been more important in some articles than the data to which they were applied. In these cases, the method of analysis and its rationale have the same epistemological status as a theory and should be presented in the introduction to the article.

And finally, if the results section is complicated or divided into several parts, you may wish to provide an overview of the section: "The results are presented in three parts. The first section presents the behavioral results for the men, followed by the parallel results for the women. The final section presents the attitudinal and physiological data for both sexes combined." But as I argue below, this kind of "process commentary" should be used very sparingly. In most cases, the prose itself should make it unnecessary.

Presenting the Findings. The general rule in reporting your findings is to give the forest first and then the trees. This is true of the results section as a whole: Begin with the central findings, and then move to more peripheral ones. It is also true within subsections: State the basic finding first, and then elaborate or qualify it as necessary. Similarly, discuss an overall measure of aggression or whatever first, and then move to its individual components. Beginning with one of your most central results, proceed as follows:

1. Remind us of the conceptual hypothesis or question you are asking: "It will be recalled that the men are expected to be more emotionally expressive than the woman." Or, "We ask, first, whether the men or the women are more emotionally expressive." Note that this is a *conceptual* statement of the hypothesis or question.
2. Remind us of the operations performed and behaviors measured: "In particular, the men should produce more tears during the showing of the film than the woman." Or, "Do the men produce more tears during the showing of the film than the women?" Note that this is an *operational* statement of the hypothesis or question.
3. Tell us the answer immediately and in English: "The answer is yes." Or, "As Table 1 reveals, men do, in fact, cry more profusely than women."

4. Now, and only now, speak to us in numbers. (Your grandmother can now skip to the next result in case she has forgotten her statistics or her reading glasses.): "Thus the men in all four conditions produced an average of 1.4 cc more tears than the women, F (1, 112) = 5.79, $p <$ .025."

5. Now you may elaborate or qualify the overall conclusion if necessary: "Only in the Father-watching condition did the men fail to produce more tears than the women, but a specific test of this effect failed to reach significance, t = 1.58, $p <$ .12."

6. End each section of the results with a summary of where things stand: "Thus, except for the father-watching condition, which will be discussed below, the hypothesis that men cry more than women in response to visually depicted grief appears to receive strong support."

7. Lead into the next section of the results with a smooth transition sentence: "Men may thus be more expressive than women in the domain of negative emotion, but are they more expressive in the domain of positive emotion? Table 2 shows they are not . . ." (Again, the "bottom line" is given immediately.) As the results section proceeds, continue to summarize and "update" the reader's store of information frequently. The reader should not have to keep looking back to retrieve the major points of your plot line.

By structuring the results section in this way, by moving from forest to trees, by announcing each result clearly in prose before wading into numbers and statistics, and by summarizing frequently, you permit a reader to decide just how much detail he or she wants to pursue at each juncture and to skip ahead to the next main point whenever that seems desirable.

Figures and Tables. Unless a set of findings can be stated in one or two numbers, results that are sufficiently important to be stressed should be accompanied by a figure or table summarizing the relevant data. The basic rule of presentation is that a reader be able to grasp your major findings *either* by reading the text *or* by looking at the figures and tables. Thus, figures and tables must be titled and labeled clearly and completely, even if that means constructing a very lengthy title or heading ("Mean number of tears produced by two affective films as a function of affect valence, subject sex, parental observation, and self-esteem"). Within the text itself, lead the reader by the hand through a table to point out the results of interest: "As shown in Column A of Table 2, men produce more tears (2.33 cc) than women (1.89 cc). . . . Of particular interest is the number of tears produced when both father and mother watch (Rows 3 and 4) . . ." Don't just wave in the general direction of the table and expect the reader to ferret out the information. For detailed information on figures and tables, see the *Publication Manual* (APA, 1983).

On Statistics. As you know, every comparison between groups or relationship between variables should be accompanied by its level of statistical significance. Otherwise, readers have no way of knowing whether the findings could have emerged by chance. But despite the importance of inferential statistics, they are not the heart of your narrative and should be subordinated to the descriptive results. Whenever possible, state a result first and then give its statistical significance, but in no case should you ever give the statistical test alone without interpreting it substantively. Do not tell us that the three-way interaction with sex, parent condition, and self-esteem was significant at the .05 level unless you tell us immediately and in English that men are less expressive than women in the negative conditions if father watches—but only for men with low self-esteem.

If your experiment utilized an analysis of variance design, your data analysis will automatically display the effects of several independent variables on a single dependent variable. If this organization is consonant with a smooth presentation of your results, lucky you. Go with it. But don't be a prisoner of ANOVA! If the narrative flows more smoothly by discussing the effects of a single independent variable on several conceptually related dependent variables tear your ANOVA results apart and reorganize them. Statistical designs are all right in their place, but you—and your prose—are master; they are slave.

Just as your method section should give readers a feel for the procedures employed, so too, the results section should give them a feel for the behavior observed. Select descriptive indices or statistics that convey the behavior of your subjects as vividly as possible. Tell us the percentage of children in your study who hit the Bobo doll or the mean number of times they did so. Remind us that a score of 3.41 on your 5-point rating scale of aggression lies between "slightly aggressive" and "moderately aggressive."

Do this even if the statistical analyses must be performed on some more indirect datum (e.g., the arcsin transform of the number of Bobo hits or the sum of three standardized aggression sources.) Display these indirect indices, too, if you wish, but give the readers' intuitions first priority. For example, in our study of trait consistency, we analyzed a standard-score index of individual consistency, but we discussed the results in terms of the more familiar correlation coefficient—on which no legitimate statistical analysis could be performed (Bem & Allen, 1974).

After you have presented your quantitative results, it is often useful to become more informal and briefly to describe the behavior of particular individuals in your study. Again, the point is not to prove something, but to add richness to your findings, to share with readers the feel of the behavior: "Indeed, two of the men used an entire box of Kleenex during the showing of the heart operation but would not pet the baby kitten owned by the secretary."

The Discussion Section

As noted earlier, the discussion section can either be combined with the results section or appear separately. In either case, it forms a cohesive narrative with the introduction, and you should expect to move materials back and forth between these two sections as you rewrite and reshape the report. Topics that are central to your story will appear in the introduction and probably again in the discussion. More peripheral topics may not be brought up at all until after the presentation of the results. The discussion is also the bottom of the hourglass-shaped format and thus proceeds from specific matters about your study to more general concerns (about methodological strategies, for example) to the broadest generalizations you wish to make. The sequence of topics is often the mirror image of the sequence in the introduction.

Begin the discussion by telling us what you have learned from the study. Open with a clear statement on the support or nonsupport of the hypotheses or the answers to the questions you first raised in the introduction. But do not simply reformulate and repeat points already summarized in the results section. Each new statement should contribute something new to the reader's understanding of the problem. What inferences can be drawn from the findings? These inferences may be at a level quite close to the data or may involve considerable abstraction, perhaps to the level of a larger theory regarding, say, emotion or sex differences. What are the theoretical, practical, or even the political implications of the results?

It is also appropriate at this point to compare your results with those reported by other investigators and to discuss possible shortcomings of your study, conditions that might limit the extent of legitimate generalization or otherwise qualify your inferences. Remind readers of the characteristics of your subject sample, the possibility that it might differ from other populations to which you might want to generalize; of specific characteristics of your methods that might have influenced the outcome; or of any other factors that might have operated to produce atypical results.

But do not dwell compulsively on every flaw! In particular, be willing to accept negative or unexpected results without a tortured attempt to explain them away. Don't make up long, involved, pretzel-shaped theories to account for every hiccup in the data. There is a -.73 correlation between the clarity of an investigator's results and the length of his or her discussion section. Don't contribute to this shameful statistic.

Ah, but suppose that, on the contrary, your results have led you to a grand new theory that injects startling clarity into your data and revolutionizes your view of the problem area. Doesn't that justify a long discussion section? No. In this case, you should write the article so that you *begin* with your new theory. As noted earlier, your task is to provide the most informative and compelling framework for your study from the opening sentence. If your new theory does that, don't wait until the discussion section to spring it on us. A journal article is not a chronology of your thought processes.

The discussion section also includes a consideration of questions that remain unanswered or that have been raised by the study itself, along with suggestions for the kinds of research that would help to answer them. In fact, suggesting further research is probably the most common way of ending a research report.

Common, but dull. The hourglass shape of the article implies that your final words should be broad general statements of near-cosmic significance, not precious details of interest only to psychologists. Thus the statement, "Further research will be needed before it is clear whether the androgyny scale should be scored as a single continuous dimension or partitioned into a 4-way typology," might well be appropriate somewhere in a discussion section, but, please, not your final farewell. In my opinion, only Montaigne was clever enough to end an article with a statement about further research. "Because [the study of motivation] is a high and hazardous undertaking, I wish fewer people would meddle with it" (1580, p. 126).

You should probably settle for more modest injunctions: "If gender schema theory has a political message, it is . . . that . . . human behaviors and personality attributes should no longer be linked with gender, and society should stop projecting gender into situations irrelevant to genitalia. The feminist prescription, then, is not that the individual be androgynous, but that the society be gender-aschematic" (S. Bem, 1985, p. 222).

But in any case, end with a bang, not a whimper.

The Title and Abstract

The title and abstract of your article permit potential readers to get a quick overview of your study and to decide if they wish to read the article itself. Titles and abstracts are also indexed and compiled in reference works and computerized databases. For this reason they should accurately reflect the content of the article and include key words that will ensure their retrieval from a database. You should compose the title and abstract after you have completed the article and have a firm view of its structure and content.

The recommended length for a title is 12 to 15 words. It should be fully explanatory when standing alone and identify the theoretical issues or the variables under investigation. Because you will not be able to mention all the features of your study in the title (or even in the abstract), you must decide which are most important. Once again, the data should guide you. For example, the most instructive findings from our fictitious study on emotional expression should determine which of the following is the most appropriate title: "Laughing versus Crying: Sex Differences in the Public Display of Positive and Negative Emotions"; "Effects of Being Observed by Parents on the Emotional Responses of Men and Women to Visual Stimuli"; "Emotional Responses to Visual Stimuli as a Function of Sex and Self-Esteem"; "Sex Differences in the Public Display of Emotion as a Function of the Observing Audience"; "Public versus Private Displays of Emotion in Men and Women."

The abstract of an empirical article should not exceed 150 words. It should contain the problem under investigation (in one sentence if possible); the subjects, specifying pertinent characteristics, such as number, type, age, sex, and species; the experimental method, including the apparatus, data-gathering procedures, and complete test names; the findings, including statistical significance levels; and the conclusion and the implications or applications.

Clearly the abstract must be very compact, and this requirement leads many inexperienced writers to make it unintelligible. Remove unnecessary words and eliminate less important details of method and results. But then let it breathe. In particular, allow yourself the space to make the problem under investigation clear to a casually browsing reader. Often you can plagiarize and abbreviate key statements from the article itself. Here is an example:

> Men are allegedly less emotionally expressive than women, but expressiveness may depend upon the situation and the specific emotion evoked. One hundred male and 100 female undergraduates were individually shown a sad or a happy movie, believing that they were being observed by one or both of their parents. Blind judges rated subjects' facial expressions, and a Lachrymeter measured their tear volume. Men cried more during the sad movie but laughed less during the happy movie than did the women (interaction, $p < .02$). However, men in the father-watching condition with low-self-esteem (Darley Self-Concept Scale) cried less than all other subjects ($p < .05$), a result consistent with Zanna's parental-role theory of emotional expression

(1952). Sex differences in emotional expression are apparently moderated by both the valence of the emotion and—for men—by self-esteem and conditions of being observed.

If the conceptual contribution of your article is more important than the supporting study, this can be reflected in the abstract by omitting experimental details and giving more space to the theoretical material. Here is the title and abstract from our *Psychological Review* article on trait consistency (Bem & Allen, 1974):

On Predicting Some of the People Some of the Time:
The Search for Cross-Situational Consistencies in Behavior

The historically recurring controversy over the existence of cross-situational consistencies in behavior is sustained by the discrepancy between our intuitions, which affirm their existence, and the research literature, which does not. It is argued that the nomothetic assumptions of the traditional research paradigm are incorrect and that by adopting some of the idiographic assumptions employed by our intuitions, higher cross-situational correlation coefficients can be obtained. A study is reported which shows it is possible to identify on a priori grounds those individuals who will be cross-situationally consistent and those who will not. It is concluded that not only must personality assessment attend to situations—as has been recently urged—but to persons as well.

REWRITING IT

For many authors revising an article is unmitigated agony. Even proofreading is painful. And so they don't. So relieved to get a draft done, they send it off to the journal thinking that they can clean up the writing after it has been accepted. Alas, that day rarely comes. Some may find solace in the belief that the manuscript probably would have been rejected even if it had been extensively revised and polished, after all, most of our journals accept only 15%–20% of all manuscripts submitted. But from my experience as an editor, I believe that the difference between the manuscripts accepted and the top 15%–20% of those rejected is frequently the difference between good and less good writing. Moral: Don't expect journal reviewers to discern your brilliance through the smog of polluted writing. Revise your manuscript. Polish it. Proofread it. *Then* submit it.

Rewriting is difficult for several reasons. First, it is difficult to edit your own writing. You will not notice ambiguities and explanatory gaps because *you* know what you meant to say and *you* understand the omitted steps. One strategy for overcoming this difficulty is to lay your manuscript aside for awhile and then return to it later when it has become less familiar. Sometimes it helps to read it aloud. But there is no substitute for practicing the art of taking the role of the nonspecialist reader, for learning to role-play grandma. As you read, ask yourself, "Have I been told yet what this concept means?" "Has the logic of this step been demonstrated?" "Would I know what the independent variable is at this point?" This is precisely the skill of the good lecturer in Psychology 100, the ability to anticipate the audience's level of understanding at each point in the presentation. Good writing is good teaching.

But because this is not easy, you should probably give a fairly polished copy of the manuscript to a friend or colleague for a critical review. (If you get a critique from two colleagues you will have simulated a trial run of a journal's review process.) The best readers are those who have themselves published in the psychological journals, but who are unfamiliar with the subject of your article. (A student from Psychology 100 would probably be too intimidated to give usefully critical feedback; grandma will be too kind.)

If your colleagues find something unclear, do not argue with them. They are right: *By definition, the writing is unclear.* Their suggestions for correcting the unclarities may be wrong, even dumb. But as unclarity detectors, readers are never wrong. Also resist the temptation simply to clarify their confusion verbally. Your colleagues don't want to offend you or appear stupid, and so they will simply mumble "oh yes, of course, of course" and apologize for not having read carefully enough. As a consequence, you will be pacified, and your next readers, the journal reviewers, will stumble over the same problem. They will not apologize; they will reject.

Rewriting is difficult for a second reason: It requires a high degree of compulsiveness and attention to detail. The probability of writing a sentence perfectly the first time is vanishingly small, and good writers rewrite nearly every sentence of an article in the course of polishing successive drafts. But even good writers differ from one another in their approach to the first draft. Some spend a long time carefully choosing each word and reshaping each sentence and paragraph as they go. Others pound out a rough draft quickly and then go back for extensive revision. Although I personally prefer the former method, I think it wastes time. For journal articles in particular, I think most authors should get the first draft done as quickly as possible without agonizing over stylistic niceties. But once it is done, compulsiveness and attention to detail become the required virtues.

And finally, rewriting is difficult because it usually means restructuring. Sometimes it is necessary to discard whole sections of an article, add new ones, go back and do more data analysis, and then totally reorganize the article just to iron out a bump in the logic of the argument. Don't get so attached to your first draft that you are unwilling to tear it apart and rebuild it. (This is why the technique of crafting each sentence of a first draft wastes time. That beautiful turn of phrase that took me 40 minutes to shape gets trashed when the article gets restructured. Worse, I get so attached to the phrase that I resist restructuring until I can find a new home for it.) A badly constructed building cannot be salvaged by brightening up the wallpaper. A badly constructed article cannot be salvaged by changing words, inverting sentences, and shuffling paragraphs.

Which brings me to the word processor. Its very virtuosity at making these cosmetic changes will tempt you to tinker endlessly, encouraging you in the illusion that you are restructuring right there in front of the monitor. Do not be fooled. You are not. A word processor—even in conjunction with a fancy "outline processor"—is not an adequate restructuring tool. Moreover, it can produce flawless, physically beautiful drafts of wretched writing, encouraging you in the illusion that they are finished manuscripts ready to be submitted. Do not be fooled. They are not. To restructure, you must print out a complete copy of each successive draft of your article; spread it out on table or floor; take pencil, scissors, and scotch tape in hand; and then, all by your low-tech self, have at it.

Got that, computer buffs? File transfer the RAM from your desk-metaphor user environment onto hard copy and then invoke a real-time cut-and-paste operation while your mouse enjoys its down time.

SOME MATTERS OF STYLE

Omit Needless Words

Virtually all experienced writers agree that any written expression that deserves to be called *vigorous writing,* whether it is a short story, an article for a professional journal, or a complete book, *is* characterized by the attribute of being succinct, *concise,* and to the point. *A sentence*—no matter where in the writing it occurs—*should contain no unnecessary* or superfluous *words,* words that stand in the way of the writer's direct expression of his or her meaning and purpose. In a very similar fashion, *a paragraph*—the basic unit of organization in English prose—should contain *no unnecessary* or superfluous *sentences,* sentences that introduce peripheral content into the writing or stray from its basic narrative line. It is in this sense that a writer is like an artist executing a drawing, and it is in this sense that a writer is like an engineer designing a machine. Good writing should be economical *for the same reason that a drawing should have no unnecessary lines, and* good writing should be streamlined in the same way that *a machine* is designed to have *no unnecessary parts,* parts that contribute little or nothing to its intended function.

This prescription to be succinct and concise is often misunderstood, and *requires* judicious application. It certainly does *not* imply *that the writer* must *make all* of *his* or her *sentences short* and choppy *or* leave out all adjectives, adverbs, and qualifiers. Nor does it mean *that he* or she must *avoid* or eliminate *all detail* from the writing *and treat his* or her *subjects only in* the barest skeleton or *outline* form. *But* the requirement does imply *that every word* committed to paper should *tell* something new to the reader and contribute in a significant and non-redundant way to the message that the writer is trying to convey.

* * *

You have just read a 303 word essay on brevity. It is not a bad first draft, but a good writer or copy editor would take its message to heart and, by crossing out all the non-italicized words, cut it by 79%. Savor the result:

> Vigorous writing is concise. A sentence should contain no unnecessary words, a paragraph no unnecessary sentences, for the same reason that a drawing should have no unnecessary lines and a machine no unnecessary parts. This requires not that the writer make all his sentences short, or that he avoid all detail and treat his subjects only in outline, but that every word tell. [63 words]

This essay on brevity was written by Strunk and White (1979, p. 23) under the heading: "Omit Needless Words." Obey their injunction, for it is the most important piece of advice in this chapter. (But ignore their use of the generic "he" and "his," about which, more later.) Journal articles should also omit needless concepts, topics, anecdotes, asides, and footnotes. Clear any underbrush that clutters your narrative. If a point seems peripheral to your main theme, remove it. If you can't bring yourself to do this, put it in a footnote. Then when you revise your manuscript, remove the footnote.

Copy editing other people's writing is good practice for improving your own. It is also less painful than editing your own and much easier than actually writing. Any piece of prose will do. Here was today's exercise for my writing class; it is part of a letter Cornell sends out to potential graduate applicants. You may wish to try your hand at it.

> Psychology is a wide field of study, and we are not equally strong in all parts of it. At present, we regard our major strengths as lying in three broadly

> defined domains in which we have many faculty, and a couple of smaller areas in which we also have appreciable resources. The three primary areas are Biopsychology, Experimental Psychology, and Personality and Social Psychology; the others are Mathematical/Differential Psychology and Experimental Psychopathology. The areas and the relevant faculty are listed below. Please note that this listing is informal; it does not imply that the listed faculty members have no other interests or can readily be fitted into predefined areas. The actual network of faculty interests and responsibilities is too subtle to be described in a letter such as this. The listing is just a rough and ready way to tell you what the Field of Psychology at Cornell is like. [149 words]

Here is a reasonable revision:

> Psychology is a wide field, and our three major strengths are Biopsychology, Experimental Psychology, and Personality and Social Psychology. We also have resources in Mathematical/Differential Psychology and Experimental Psychopathology. The following list of faculty within areas provides a rough guide to the Field of Psychology at Cornell. Faculty interests are broader than this list implies, however, and do not always neatly fit the predefined areas. [66 words, a savings of 56%]

To maintain the vigor of your prose, try to spend at least 15 minutes each day omitting needless words. Your goal should be to reach at least 30% of all words encountered. (Copy edited versions of this chapter will be returned unopened.)

Avoid Process Comments

Expository writing fails its mission if it diverts the reader's attention to itself and away from the subject; the process of writing should be transparent to the reader. In particular, the prose itself should direct the flow of the narrative without requiring you to play tour guide by commenting on it. Don't say: "Now that I have discussed the three theories of emotion, we can turn to the empirical work on each of them. I will begin with the psychoanalytic account of affect . . ." Instead, move directly from your discussion of the theories into the literature review with a simple transition sentence like, "Each of these three theories has been tested empirically. Thus, the psychoanalytic account of affect has received support in studies that . . ." Don't say: "Now that we have seen the results for negative affect, we are in a position to examine men's and women's emotional expression in the realm of positive affect. The relevant data are presented in Table 2 . . ." Instead use a transition sentence that simultaneously summarizes and moves the story along: "Men may thus be more expressive than women in the domain of negative emotion, but are they also more expressive in the domain of positive emotion? Table 2 shows that they are not . . ."

If you feel the need to make process comments in order to keep the reader on the narrative path, then your plot line is probably already too cluttered, the writing insufficiently linear. Process comments will only oppress the prose further. Instead, copy edit. Omit needless words; don't add them!

Use Repetitive and Parallel Construction

Inexperienced writers often substitute synonyms for recurring words and vary their sentence structure in the mistaken belief that this is more creative, stylish, and interesting. Instead of using repetition and parallel construction, as in "Men may be more expressive than women in the domain of negative emotion, but they are not more expressive in the domain of positive emotion," they attempt to be more creative: "Men may be more expressive than women in the domain of negative emotion, but it is not true that they are more willing and able to display the more cheerful affects."

Such creativity is hardly more interesting, but it is certainly more confusing. In scientific communication, it can be deadly. When an author uses different words to refer to the same concept in a technical article—where accuracy is paramount—readers will justifiably wonder if different meanings are implied. This particular example is not disastrous, and most readers will be unaware that their understanding flickered momentarily when the prose hit a bump. But consider the cognitive burden carried by readers who must hack through this "creative" jungle: "The high-dissonance subjects were paid a small sum of money while being given a free choice of whether or not to participate, whereas the participants we randomly assigned to the large-incentive treatment (the low-dissonance condition) were not offered the opportunity to refuse." This author should have written "High-dissonance subjects were paid a small sum of money and were not required to participate; low-dissonance subjects were paid a large sum of money and were required to participate." The wording and grammatical structure of the two clauses are held rigidly parallel; only the variables vary. Repetition and parallel construction are among the most effective servants of clarity. Don't be creative, be clear.

Repetition and parallel construction also serve clarity at a larger level of organization. By providing the reader with distinctive guideposts to the structure of the prose, they can diminish or eliminate the need for process comments. Here, for example, are the opening sentences from three of the paragraphs in the earlier section on rewriting:

2nd paragraph: "Rewriting is difficult for several reasons. First . . ."
5th paragraph: "Rewriting is difficult for a second reason:"
6th paragraph: "And finally, rewriting is difficult because it . . ."

If I had substituted synonyms for the recurring words or varied the grammatical structure of these opening sentences, their guiding function would have been lost, the reader's sense of the section's organization blurred.

And finally, repetition and parallel construction can serve style and creativity as well as clarity. They can provide rhythm and punch: "A sentence should contain no unnecessary words, a paragraph no unnecessary sentences for the same reason that a drawing should have no unnecessary lines and a machine no unnecessary parts." They can establish metaphor: "A badly constructed building cannot be salvaged by brightening up the wallpaper. A badly constructed article cannot be salvaged by changing words, inverting sentences, and shuffling paragraphs." They can add humor: "The word processor encourages you in the illusion that you are restructuring. Do not be fooled. You are not. The word processor encourages you in the illusion that your drafts are finished manuscripts. Do not be fooled. They are not."

Jargon

Jargon is the specialized vocabulary of a discipline, and it serves a number of legitimate functions in scientific communication. A specialized term may be more general, more precise, or freer of surplus meaning than any natural language equivalent (e.g., the term *disposition* encompasses, and hence is more general than, beliefs, attitudes, moods, and personality attributes; *reinforcement* is more precise and freer of surplus meaning than *reward*). And the technical vocabulary often makes an important conceptual distinction not apprehended by the layperson's vocabulary (e.g., genotype versus phenotype).

But if a jargon term does not satisfy any of these criteria, opt for English. Much of our jargon has become second-nature to us and serves only to muddy our prose for the general reader. (I once had to interrogate an author at length to learn that a prison program for "strengthening the executives functions of the ego" actually taught prisoners how to fill out job applications.) And unless the jargon term is extremely well known (e.g., reinforcement), it should be defined—explicitly, implicitly, or by example—the first time it is introduced. (See the sample opening statements earlier in this chapter for ways to do this.)

Voice and Self-Reference

In the past, scientific writers used the passive voice almost exclusively and referred to themselves in the third person: "This experiment was designed by the authors to test . . ." This practice produces lifeless prose and is no longer the norm. Use the active voice unless style or content dictates otherwise; and, in general, keep self-reference to a minimum. Remember that you are not the subject of your article. You should not refer to yourself as "the author" or "the investigator." (You may refer to "the experimenter" in the method section, however, even if that happens to be you; the experimenter *is* part of the subject under discussion there.) Do not refer to yourself as "we" unless there really are two or more of you. You may refer to yourself as "I," but do so sparingly. It tends to distract the reader from the topic, and it is better to remain in the background. Leave the reader in the background, too. Don't say, "The reader will find it hard to believe that . . ." or "You will be surprised to learn . . ." (This chapter violates the rule because you and your prose *are* the subject.)

It is permissible to refer to yourself and the reader as "we" in some contexts: "We can see in Table 1 that most of the tears . . ." "In everyday life, of course, we overestimate the degree to which . . ." And you may also refer to the reader indirectly in imperative, "you-understood" sentences: "Consider, first, the results for women." "Note particularly the difference between the means in Table 1."

Tense

Use the past tense when reporting the previous research of others ("Bandura reported . . ."), how you conducted your study ("Observers were posted behind . . ."), and specific past behaviors of your subjects ("Two of the men talked . . ."). Use the present tense for results currently in front of the reader ("As Table 2 shows, the negative film is more effective . . .") and for conclusions that are more general than the specific results ("Positive emotions, then, are more easily expressed when . . .")

Gender

Most publishers, including the American Psychological Association, now require authors to avoid language that reinforces sex stereotypes and common assumptions about sex roles. The most awkward problems arise from the common use of masculine nouns and pronouns when the content refers to both sexes. The generic use of "man," "he," "his," and "him" to refer to both sexes is not only misleading in many instances, but research shows that readers think of male persons when these forms are used (Martyna, 1978). Sometimes the results are not only sexist, but humorous in their naive androcentrism: "Man's vital needs include food, water, and access to females" (Quoted in Martyna, 1978).

Unfortunately, the language has not kept pace with this new awareness, and the available alternatives are not wholly satisfactory. (Which is why Strunk and White continue to advocate the use of the generic masculine pronouns. You may agree, but journal editors will overrule you.) In most contexts, the simplest alternative is the use of the plural. Instead of saying, "The individual who displays prejudice in his personal relations . . . ," say "Individuals who display prejudice in their personal relations are . . ." If it is stylistically important to focus on the single individual, the use of "he or she," "him or her," and so forth is acceptable but clumsy if used very often. Alternatives like he/she or s/he are distracting, unpronounceable, and grate on the eye. Don't use them. Eventually our society might adopt one of the neutral forms currently being suggested (e.g., "e" or "tey"), but none of them has yet won acceptance.

You may find it instructive to review how I have dealt with the pronoun problem in this chapter. In particular, note the many references to the "reader" or "readers." Sometimes the plural worked fine (e.g., "Don't plunge readers into the middle of your problem. Take the time to lead them . . ."), but in other instances the imagery of the sentence required the stylistic use of the singular (e.g., "Lead the reader by the hand through a table . . ."). In these cases, I have usually sought ways of wording the sentence in order to keep the awkward "he or she" construction to a minimum.

Stylistic matters aside, however, you must be accurate in your use of pronouns when you describe your research or that of others. Readers must be explicitly told the sex of experimenters, observers, and subjects. When referring to males, use male pronouns; when referring to females, use female pronouns. (See, for example, the earlier description of the Festinger-Carlsmith study, which used male subjects.) Under no circumstances should you omit or hide sex identity in a misguided attempt to be unbiased.

The problems of gender reference become easier when we move away from pronouns. Words like man and mankind are easily replaced by terms like people and humanity. Instead of manning projects, we can staff them. The federal government has already desexed occupational titles so that we have letter carriers rather then mailmen; in private industry we have flight attendants rather than stewardesses. And in life, children need nurturing or parenting, not just mothering. In all these cases, you will find it easy to discover the appropriate sex-neutral term if you think of the activity rather than the person doing it.

Next, watch out for the plain old stereotyping. The author who asserts that "research scientists often neglect their wives" fails to acknowledge that women as well as men are research scientists. If the author meant specifically male research scientists, he (she?) should have said so. Do not talk about ambitious men and aggressive women or cautious men and timid women if the use of different adjectives denotes not different behaviors on the part of men and women but your stereotyped interpretation of those behaviors. Don't make stereotyped assumptions about marital sex roles by saying that "The client's husband lets her teach part-time" if all you know is that the client teaches part-time. If the bias is not yours but someone else's, let the writing make that clear: "The client's husband 'lets' her teach part-time." "The husband says he 'lets' the client teach part-time." "The client says her husband lets her teach part-time." "The client says sarcastically that her husband 'lets' her teach part-time." The client and her husband are allowed to say such things. You are not.

And finally, select examples with care. Beware of your assumptions about the sex of doctors, homemakers, nurses, and so forth. Why not: "The athlete who believes in her ability to succeed . . ."? Let our writing promote the view that woman's vital needs are the same as man's: food, water, and access to equality.

For additional information, see Section 2.12 of the *Publication Manual,* "Guidelines for Nonsexist Language in APA Journals" (APA, 1983, pp. 43–49). Do not see Strunk and White!

Common Errors of Grammar and Usage

The following errors seem to me to be the most frequent in journal writing (listed alphabetically):

Compared with versus *Compared to.* Similar orders of things are compared *with* one another; different orders of things are compared *to* one another: "Let me not compare thee *with* previous lovers I have had; rather, let me compare thee *to* a summer's day." "Mischel's articles are often compared *with* Bandura's articles; Bem's articles are often compared *to* Mozart's sonatas."

Data. The word *data* is plural: "Analyze those data thoroughly."

Different from versus *Different than.* The first is correct, the second, incorrect (although, alas for us purists, very common and gaining respectability). The confusion arises because *than* correctly follows comparative adjectives. Thus you are correct to suppose that life is more *than* psychology, that living a good life is harder in many respects *than* writing a good article, and that living well requires broader skills *than* does writing well. Just remember that life is different *from* psychology, that living a good life is different in many respects *from* writing a good article, and that living well requires skills different *from* those required for writing well.

None, No one. These words are singular: "None of them is likely to obtain data that are more convincing."

Since versus *Because.* *Since* means "after that." It cannot substitute for *because*. Wrong: "Since the study of motivation is a high and hazardous undertaking, I wish fewer people would meddle with it." Right: "Because the study of motivation is a high and hazardous undertaking, I wish fewer people would meddle with it." Ambiguous: "Since I read Montaigne, I have been tempted to abandon the study of motivation." This last case is correct if the writer is using *since* in the temporal sense: "Ever since reading Montaigne, I have been tempted . . ." It is incorrect if the writer means *because*.

That versus *Which.* *That* clauses (called restrictive) are essential to the meaning of the sentence; *which* clauses (called nonrestrictive) merely add further information. The following example illustrates the correct use of both words: "Dissonance theory, *which* has received major attention, is one of the theories *that* postulates a motivational process. Thus, if a person holds two cognitions *that* are inconsistent . . ." Most *which's* in journal writing are incorrect. You should go on a *which* hunt in your own manuscripts and turn most of them into *that's*.

While versus *Although, But, Whereas.* *While* means "at the same time" and in most cases cannot substitute for these other words. Wrong: "While inferential statistics are important, descriptive statistics are the heart of your narrative." Right: "Although inferential statistics are important, descriptive statistics are the heart of your narrative." Or, "Inferential statistics are important, but descriptive statistics are the heart of your narrative." Wrong: "While I like personality traits, Mischel prefers a social learning approach." Right: "Whereas I like personality traits, Mischel prefers a social learning approach." Interestingly, the following usage is correct: "While I like personality traits, I find merit in Mischel's social learning approach." This can be seen by substituting "at the same time" for "while": "I like personality traits; at the same time, I find merit in Mischel's social learning approach."

Beyond Publication

In writing this chapter, I have presumed that your pressing pragmatic purpose is to transform your studies into publishable—nay, published—prose. But let your grander goal be to gift that prose with the effortless grace and supple simplicity of a Mozart sonata. This guiding metaphor may not turn all your studies into publications—even Mozart died a pauper—but it will turn even your sow's ears into vinyl purses.

REFERENCES

American Psychological Association. (1983). *Publication manual* (3rd ed.). Washington, DC: Author.

Bem, D. J., & Allen, A. (1974). Predicting some of the people some of the time: The search for cross-situational consistencies in behavior. *Psychological Review, 81,* 506–520.

Bem, S. L. (1985). Androgyny and gender schema theory: A conceptual and empirical integration. In T. B. Sonderegger (Ed.), *Nebraska symposium on motivation 1984: The psychology of gender* (pp. 179–226). Lincoln: University of Nebraska Press.

Festinger, L. A. (1957). *A theory of cognitive dissonance*. Stanford: Stanford University Press.

Festinger, L., & Carlsmith, J. M. (1959). Cognitive consequences of forced compliance. *Journal of Personality and Social Psychology, 58,* 203–210.

Martyna, W. (1978). What does "He" mean? *Journal of Communication, 28,* 131–138.

Montaigne, Michel de. (1580/1943). Of the inconsistency of our actions. In D. M. Frame (Translator), *Selected essays*. Roslyn, NY: Walter J. Black.

Strunk, W., Jr., & White, E. B. (1979). *The elements of style* (3rd ed.). New York: Macmillan.

III ADVICE FOR SOCIAL SCIENTISTS IN NONACADEMIC SETTINGS

9
AN INCOMPLEAT GUIDE TO WORKING AS A NONACADEMIC RESEARCHER

William DeJong
Education Development Center

Leonard Saxe
Boston University

Izak Walton's (1653/1931) *The Compleat Angler* opened the world of sport fishing to many who would not have otherwise recognized its attractions as a pastime. In a similar way, Hershoff's (1956) more recent "compleat" book described the joys of small sailing vessels and how one can make do with little and gain tremendous enjoyment. These two books, by illuminating the pleasures of a simpler life, provide a useful message for readers caught up in the grind of modern technological society.

For us as social psychologists, the present chapter concerns a similar return to basics. Social psychology had its origins in applied research that attempted to come to grips intellectually with important practical problems. But the development of social psychology as a separate academic discipline, which began just over 25 years ago, moved the field away from applied research. Now, as more social psychologists show a renewed interest in applied work, new Ph.D.'s are increasingly finding jobs in nonacademic settings (Pion & Lipsey, 1984). Work in these settings involves, to some extent, a return to basics and, as such, has much to recommend it.

In this chapter, we describe both the pleasures and pains of working as researchers outside academia. Unfortunately, we are not able to describe the world of nonacademic research with quite the same literary flair shown by Walton and Hershoff. (Nonacademic research, unlike fishing and sailing, is not appreciated for its recuperative powers, nor does it lend itself easily to metaphorical description.) Nevertheless, we hope that our readers will be tempted by what follows to travel beyond their present boundaries and that they will be better prepared to navigate and even to enjoy the terrain when they arrive.

NONACADEMIC RESEARCH CAREERS

Many doctoral students in psychology enter graduate school in pursuit of an academic career. It is, of course, a career that has much to offer—the opportunity to contribute to a specialized area of knowledge; the excitement of instructing students in the methods and theories of psychology; continual exposure to new ideas; the freedom to define an intellectual direction. At best, faculty salaries are modest, but there are offsetting advantages—prestige; a stimulating (and perhaps uncommonly beautiful) work environment; few rigidly imposed job requirements; day-to-day variety; flexible hours. And there is security: once professors are tenured, they enjoy a level of job security rivaled only by U.S. postal workers.

The goal of an academic career is one that few of today's doctoral students will realize, however, for they are caught in a demographic "squeeze play." On the one hand, the number of newly matriculated freshmen at the nation's universities is expected to continue to decline well into the 1990s. On the other hand, many academic faculties are presently 60% to 70% tenured. Large numbers of professors were tenured in the late 1960s or early 1970s when college enrollments were at a peak, and these professors are twenty or more years away from retirement. If for no other reason, freshly minted Ph.D.'s who want to conduct research will have to consider working in nonacademic settings.

We are confident, however, that as more and more psychologists-in-training consider nonacademic research careers, they will discover that such work holds its own attractions. Although academic research is primarily valued for its contribution to theory, many academicians are discouraged that their work is seldom, if ever, applied to real-world problems. Many psychologists who have made the transition to nonacademic research find it exhilarating to be involved in large-scale projects that can affect corporate or government policy.[1] Additionally, many psychologists prefer collaborative work and find the individualism imposed by academia to be stifling. In contrast, research work in nonacademic settings almost always demands a team approach.

There are a number of nonacademic settings in which research psychologists presently work—for example, contract research firms or nonprofit "think-tanks" that specialize in program evaluation and policy analysis; research and development ("R & D") departments within large corporations; marketing research or management consulting firms. In some cases, psychologists have specialized knowledge that these organizations find attractive. But even if that is not the case, research psychologists typically possess an impressive array of skills that can be readily applied to nonlaboratory research, policy analysis, or consulting work.

A complete description of the types of work that research psychologists can do in nonacademic settings would require its own chapter. We think, however, that our own work amply illustrates the broad range of what nonacademic researchers can do.

In 1979, after only one year at Brandeis University, DeJong abandoned his tenure-track job to work at Abt Associates, a large contract research firm in Cambridge, Massachusetts, that specializes in policy analysis and evaluation research for the Federal government. Working in the company's criminal justice division, DeJong managed a large contract with the National Institute of Justice (NIJ) for its "exemplary projects" program. In helping NIJ identify model programs, and during other work done for Abt, he evaluated a wide range of criminal justice programs, including small claims mediation and arbitration, neighborhood crime prevention, child sexual abuse prevention and treatment, police stress, and others. DeJong presently works as a research associate for the Education Development Center (EDC), where he is evaluating patient education strategies in public venereal disease clinics and the use of microcomputer text-editor software in the teaching of composition to learning-disabled elementary school children.

Saxe holds a faculty position at Boston University in an applied social psychology program. Thus, the bulk of his applied research—initially evaluation research in health care settings and, more recently, policy research for the U.S. Congress (Saxe & Dougherty, 1985)—has been conducted within a traditional academic department. In 1979, Saxe received a Congressional Fellowship from the Office of Technology Assessment (OTA). Working as a full-time staff member at OTA for one year, and then as a consultant, Saxe developed reports on the cost-effectiveness of psychotherapy, the treatment of alcoholism, and the scientific validity of polygraph testing. Each of these studies involved synthesizing large literatures, developing a conceptual scheme to integrate information, and eventually testifying before Congressional committees about study results.

Reflecting on our nonacademic work, three points stand out. First, both of us have contributed to work across a wide range of content areas. As we explain later in this chapter, this diversity of experience is typical in nonacademic settings. Second, the general perspective we have as social psychologists (Saxe, 1983) and the skills we have in framing conceptual issues, organizing research literatures, developing research programs, conducting data analysis, and writing—skills that were honed during graduate school and our early years in academia—have served us well in this new arena. Third, we enjoy what we do. Certainly, we encounter frustrations in doing nonacademic research, and some of these are described later in this chapter. Despite them, however, we find our work to be intellectually challenging and satisfying. And, yes, the pay can be better than in academia.

Although we see many advantages to working in nonacademic settings, we must point to one key disadvantage: in such settings, researchers must frequently sacrifice their individual autonomy and must sometimes relinquish control over their work. This aspect of nonacademic work demands personal adjustment by every researcher who ventures outside academia. Unfortunately, some never do adjust, and they find that the inability to exercise complete control over their work life makes them feel disaffected and even alienated from their work.

This confirms for us that most psychology students are ill-prepared to work effectively in nonacademic settings. Their graduate training normally teaches them to conduct research as solitary scholars and to believe that the exercise of total control is the *sine qua non* of being a good researcher. Of course, scholarly work in psychology is subject to informal methods of control (e.g., grant review panels, journal editorial policies), so it is an overstatement to say that university scholars have complete freedom. But within the boundaries defined by a discipline's *zeitgeist,* that freedom certainly exists. Outside academia, it seldom does. Graduate programs must do a better job of preparing their students for this reality.

In the next section, we describe more fully how work is accomplished in nonacademic settings, focusing on the differences between those settings and academia. We offer you fair warning: the constraints on autonomy outside academia are real. Following that, we outline the skills that graduate students in psychology can develop to get and keep a job outside academia. We sincerely believe that psychology Ph.D.'s with the right mix of skills can work successfully, even thrive, as evaluation researchers, policy analysts, or consultants in the nonacademic world.

NONACADEMIC RESEARCH SETTINGS

Why does research work in nonacademic settings constrain the autonomy of individual researchers? Many threats to autonomy are endemic to the work itself or to the organizational context in which the work is performed. Quite simply, nonacademic research typically involves several other people, each with a stake in its outcome—those who sponsor the work, fellow members of the research team, and supervisors for the research organization who manage the staff and oversee the research. As we describe how each of these three groups can affect individual researchers, remember that not every constraint operates universally. Just as there is no typical university, there is no typical nonacademic research setting.[2]

Research Sponsors

Much of the work done in nonacademic settings is "contract research" for federal, state, or local government agencies. An important feature of such research is that the contract researchers work in the service of the funding agency, often referred to as the "client." A second important consideration is that the research sponsor is paying for policy recommendations that the agency can consider, not for basic knowledge or theory. Although distinctions between basic knowledge and application are often difficult to make, researchers who conduct nonacademic research no longer assess the worth of their work solely in terms of its "academic contribution," but instead focus on its utility, often to a particular client.

The research sponsor usually defines what work is to be done by means of a "request for proposals" (RFP). At a minimum, the RFP specifies what research issues the agency wants explored. Beyond that, the RFP sometimes lists what hypotheses are to be tested, independent and dependent variables, the methodology to be used, the work schedule, and the format for the final report. Research organizations (and university groups) are invited to submit a proposal that describes how they would accomplish the research.

Once the research sponsor selects a particular proposal, representatives from both the agency and the research organization meet to negotiate a contract that will specify exactly what "service" will be delivered. Even when the RFP is fairly explicit, various approaches to the work are possible, so any differences of opinion between the funding agency and the research organization must be resolved at this time. If a compromise satisfactory to the researchers cannot be reached, the research organization, because of its concern about bringing in contract revenue, will feel pressured to capitulate to the contract terms dictated by the sponsor. At the same time, the funding agency, because of its own need for a quick resolution of these negotiations, will often agree to contract terms suggested by the research organization that are not to the agency's advantage.

Even after the contract is signed, the funding agency's day-to-day influence on the project staff continues. The funder will sometimes have a stake in a certain research outcome or a set of policy recommendations. When this is the case, the conduct of the research and the description and interpretation of results may be affected. Pressure from the sponsor is not always easily resisted, especially when the research organization is eager to secure future work from the agency. Thus, not only are researchers working in the service of their client, but they may sometimes find themselves in the service of a particular position held by that client.

The value of government-sponsored research is defined in a political environment, and an important feature of that environment is its volatility. As a result, the funder may require changes in the project design or work schedule at any time. Of greater concern is that, because of changes in the political winds, a research project's constituency within the sponsoring agency may disappear, which can result in project termination. It can also mean that a final report or other research products may be accepted without comment and shelved. In either case, the project can be stripped of meaning by forces outside the researchers' control.

A research sponsor can impose other constraints. Sometimes, for example, the deadline imposed on the work is unrealistically tight. Obviously, severe time pressures necessarily diminish the scope of inquiry. The researchers may also have to rush their work or put in overtime to meet the deadline, both of which can affect the quality of work and the researchers' morale. Nevertheless, even if it is widely agreed that the research would be enhanced, the agency's immediate need for information and recommendations (or bureaucratic inflexibility) may prevent the agency's project monitor from changing the deadline.

Limited research budgets can also introduce significant constraints. To ensure that work is accomplished under budget, research organizations must impose tight budgetary controls and contract review procedures. Because of this, and because researchers' salaries come primarily from the contracts on which they work (referred to as "soft money," as opposed to teaching salaries which are "hard money"), there must be a direct means-end relationship between their activities and the service or product purchased by the client. Each hour of the researchers' time must be focused on the task at hand. With this "product-orientation," free-floating exploration of ideas and alternative approaches or a careful examination of the research literature may be curtailed. Researchers, moreover, may have little time available for accumulating new knowledge or skills.

Because contract funds can be terminated at the convenience of the research sponsor, researchers must work according to that sponsor's specifications. Researchers, however, are not without countervailing power. First, they derive power from their expertise. Rosenblum and McGillis (1979) note that researchers have greater power when an agency must act quickly and when the researchers themselves are nationally recognized experts. Second, especially after work is underway, the agency's project monitor has a stake in making the selection of a particular research organization appear wise. There may also be enormous financial costs involved in cancelling a contract. Nevertheless, research organizations must look beyond the project at hand to future contracts, and because of this, there is no doubt where the ultimate power lies.

Research work for marketing research firms, management consulting firms, or R & D departments shares a number of important features with government contract research. The nature of the research project is defined by the research sponsor, which can be either the parent company or an outside client. Again, ultimate control over the project rests with those who are paying for it. In addition, the parent company or the outside client must respond to the demands of the marketplace, which can also create a volatile environment in which to conduct research. Time pressures and budgetary constraints can be severe, which sometimes forces researchers to sacrifice quality for the sake of expediency.

Grant support. When research work is funded by outside grants rather than contracts, many fewer constraints are placed on the researchers. For most grants, the research sponsor, whether it is a government agency, a corporation, or a foundation, identifies general priority areas, but then relies on individual researchers or firms to specify a research question, the independent and dependent variables, and the experimental methods. A review panel is then used to select those proposals that hold the greatest promise.

Grants are relatively open-ended agreements. A certain line of research is funded, and the researchers' ability to garner further support depends on successful completion of that work. But there is also wide recognition that the researchers themselves will modify the work plan as needed. Planned studies may prove to be infeasible, for example, or early work may take the research in unexpected directions. In short, the research sponsor is primarily concerned that the research be done well and is less likely to be invested in a particular research outcome or set of policy recommendations. Thus, even in nonacademic settings, grant funding can provide individual researchers with considerable autonomy.

Although grant awards are most often used to fund "basic research," some government agencies are using such awards to fund work that will be directly useful to policymakers. The primary motive for this is the agencies' hope of saving money, for with grants, research organizations cannot charge a percentage fee (i.e., a built-in profit) on top of overhead. Proposal requests for such grants can be quite explicit about what work is needed, as is usually the case with contract RFPs.

Research Teams

Research work in nonacademic settings normally requires a team approach, either because a large block of work must be accomplished under severe time constraints, which a solitary researcher cannot complete successfully, or because a project may call for skills or specialized knowledge beyond the capabilities of a single researcher. To conduct this work, research organizations assemble teams of researchers (along with a phalanx of research assistants, data coders, and secretaries) to work on particular projects. Once projects are finished, teams are disassembled, and reconfigured teams are brought together to meet the demands of new projects.

From the standpoint of individual researchers, there are four principal advantages to being part of a research team: (1) The quality of work may be enhanced when there are several contributors of varied backgrounds and an interchange of ideas among them. It should be noted, however, that the value of so-called interdisciplinary teams is sometimes oversold; differences in orientation may occasionally be so severe that work is impeded. (2) Exposure to others' knowledge, skills, and perspective can expand a reseacher's own expertise. (3) Feedback from members of the research team is fairly immediate. (4) For many researchers, working closely with other people can be more enjoyable than working in isolation.

For a researcher trained in the individualistic tradition of academia, however, being part of a team can present difficulties:

1. Both the research design and interpretation of results may be a compromise among team members. As part of a team, individual researchers may have to accept decisions that they personally dislike.

2. Members' interdependence can result in several researchers being held up in their work while they wait for someone else's to be completed. This is not merely an issue of individual competence; unless the research project is exceptionally large, most team members may also be involved with other projects that present conflicting work demands. Interdependence also increases the urgency of completing work on time, thus contributing to the "product-orientation" that researchers in nonacademic settings sometimes develop.

3. Project directors' power to exercise control over their research staffs varies across organizations. In some settings, a project director may be forced to take on or retain staff members who are not ideally suited for

the project or who create dissension among other team members. Under such circumstances, when one member of the team fails to complete an assignment, the other researchers, seeking to preserve both the integrity of the project and their own reputations, may be forced to carry that person's workload.

Preference for generalists. To respond to changing needs of funding agencies, research organizations must have flexible work forces. To achieve this flexibility, the organizations have two options. One is to hire specialists who are well-suited to current work, but who may have to be replaced by other specialists when work demands change. The second option is to hire generalists who can easily move from subject area to subject area and are willing to do so. Because RFPs allow only a short time to assemble research teams and submit bids, and because of the costs involved in hiring and training new personnel, the second option is usually chosen. As a result, when hiring new staff, nonacademic organizations often place a premium on general abilities rather than on specialized knowledge or training.

Once hired, most researchers feel pressured to remain generalists. For those with certain skills (e.g., data management and analysis, writing), enough projects may be available to allow them to specialize and still have job security. Others may get involved in a subject area of long-term interest to research sponsors. For many researchers, however, this will not be possible; if it is important to them to acquire cumulative knowledge or specialized skills, this will be a source of frustration.

Research organizations' preference for generalists can create additional problems for individual researchers. First, supervisors may see researchers as "interchangeable parts" and reassign them to projects without consideration of their interests or their personal investment in ongoing work. Second, building a knowledge-based reputation requires specialization, and the inability to create that base may diminish researchers' ability to re-enter academia or to generate independent grant support.

Certain R & D departments may also prefer generalists over specialists. If the parent company operates in a fast-changing market, such as the computer industry, there is a strong need for generalists who can quickly understand new areas and contribute to a research program. Specialists can be hired or trained, but the company then runs the risk of having staff whose skills are rendered obsolete by changes in the marketplace.

Research Organizations

A nonacademic research organization operates as a business—whether it is designed to produce profits for stockholders, is nonprofit, or is part of a larger corporation—and researchers are employees of that business. Individual researchers in nonacademic settings are not independent agents, meaning that they must subordinate their interests, needs, or preferences to the needs of the research organization. This manifests itself in several ways:

1. Within an organization, researchers may not receive individual recognition for their contribution to a research project. One reason, of course, is that the researchers work in teams, and individual contributions may not be easily identified. If there is a single individual who does become identified with a project, it is normally the project director, even if that person did not conduct the research work, but only administered the project.

2. Publications may carry the name of the research organization or the funding agency, rather than the names of the researchers responsible for the work. Even if the researchers are identified on the title page of the publication, press releases from the research organization or the funding agency often fail to credit individuals for their contribution.

3. A research organization may prohibit employees from publishing book chapters or journal articles without the express consent of the firm's leadership or a review committee. This policy is designed to protect the company's proprietary interests and to maintain the image of the company or its clients. Although funding agencies rarely make this constraint explicit, they can make publication of unfavorable findings difficult and may even hold proprietary claim to data generated by the project.

4. Research organizations may expect staff, including senior researchers, to be in their offices during normal business hours. Working at home or in a library may be actively discouraged, both to monitor better the researchers' work and to have staff available to deal with unexpected emergencies.

5. Most large research organizations use centralized planning to decide what "research markets" to concentrate on. Because financial and human resources are limited, individual researchers can seldom respond to RFPs that fall outside that plan. In other words, whether certain work will be pursued is an institutional decision, not an individual decision. If researchers develop interests in areas that fall outside the plan, they must convince their superiors that the chances of financial payoff are high. Companies vary, of course, in how much this kind of individual initiative is encouraged. It should also be noted that because research organizations take an institutional view, researchers are sometimes required to help write proposals for research on which they themselves will not work.

Impact of supervisors. A critical feature of nonacademic research firms is the tremendous impact of supervisors on researchers' work life.

Of course, in academia there are autocratic department chairs who greatly affect the work lives of their colleagues through decisions on laboratory and office space, teaching assignments, salaries, and so on. But in nonacademic research settings, the supervisors' influence is necessarily more pervasive.

In some research organizations, project directors are given responsibility for staffing their projects. But in many others, upper-level managers will make these assignments. From the standpoint of individual researchers, such assignments are not always made rationally: researchers may not be allowed to follow up on previous work; they may be assigned to projects for which they have no interest or direct training, including nonresearch work (e.g., software development, product or systems design); or they may be frequently reassigned. As noted before, these problems are exacerbated when supervisors view researchers as interchangeable parts.

Supervisors also manage their research organization's relationships with outside funding agencies, both to protect the organization's reputation and to attract new projects. Because of this focus, communications between supervisors and research staff often center around deadlines and money instead of the work itself. In extreme cases, supervisors may even come to view the work only as a vehicle for generating revenue. Given their different emphases, clashes between researchers and supervisors are, perhaps, inevitable.

Supervisors must "sign off" on work before it is submitted to a client. In general, supervision is high because the client has purchased a service from the research organization, not the individual researchers, and the organization's reputation is at stake. Actual quality control, however, is uneven. Supervisors often do not have the technical skills or the information necessary to evaluate the researchers' work critically, or pressing deadlines may prevent a strict enforcement of standards. But there can also be differences of opinion between supervisors and researchers over what constitutes acceptable work. Because of their focus on the financial health of the organization, supervisors may be tempted to judge the quality of work only in terms of what will please the client.

The bureaucracy within a research organization also makes demands on individual researchers. Project directors are asked to spell out (and continually revise) which staff will do what, when, and for how much money. The organization's need for this information to plan staffing needs and to make revenue projections may produce rigidity in the conduct of the research beyond whatever limitations are caused by the overall project budget. In addition, project directors may be pressured to spend contract funds quickly in order to generate overhead for the company. It should also be noted that a research organization with a large bureaucracy may have overhead rates that make it noncompetitive for certain work that may be of interest to individual researchers.

A final note: Although nonacademic researchers more clearly have a business orientation, we are convinced that sharpened competition for available research funds and tighter university budgets will push more faculty to compete with and therefore talk like their nonacademic brethren. Both at Abt Associates and EDC, DeJong has been a frequent participant in business planning meetings. But Saxe, who is still based at Boston University, finds he is attending more and more meetings where decisions to develop and submit research proposals are based on allowable overhead rates and other financial considerations, not merely researchers' interest in the work.

NONACADEMIC RESEARCH SKILLS

Psychologists trained by academicians who themselves have never worked in nonacademic environments are usually ill-prepared for working outside academia. In fact, based on our description of nonacademic research organizations, some students might conclude that these organizations are hostile settings for academically trained researchers and therefore choose to avoid them. But the answer is not to avoid such settings; rather, it is to develop the interpersonal and intellectual skills that those settings require. These skills are partly a matter of individual temperament or native ability, but they can also be practiced or shaped through work experience.

We have described below a number of such skills, ranging from interpersonal effectiveness and communication skills to the ability to meet deadlines and to function as a member of a large team. Of course, while these skills are needed for survival in applied settings, they would also prove helpful in coping with the ways and means of traditional academic institutions.

Personal Skills

As we noted previously, working on applied research involves complex relationships with research sponsors and supervisors and among members of research teams. The ability to manage these relationships is crucial to working effectively in an applied research organization and to conducting good research.

Interpersonal skills. To put it simply, researchers in nonacademic settings must be able to get along with co-workers, subordinates, supervisors, and actual or potential research clients. The range of such relationships is probably no different than that found in academia, but the seriousness with which they are taken in the applied world is far greater. Researchers may be evaluated for raises, or even for continuation of employment, on the basis of their ability to manage relationships with others.

There are several reasons for the importance attached to this skill. One is the extensive use of research teams in nonacademic settings. Another is that applied research work is often done under severe time pressures. Norms and expectations also play an important role. Academics are given a fair amount of "idiosyncrasy credit"; indeed, they may even be expected to behave in clumsy and inefficient ways. Although interpersonal awkwardness may be less bothersome in academia, it is little tolerated in research organizations that depend for their existence on good relationships with government funding agencies, corporations, or foundations.

Both of us have learned the hard way about the importance of interpersonal skills outside academia. A dissatisfied project monitor once asked DeJong to review a preliminary draft of a policy brief being prepared by one of DeJong's supervisors. Without hesitation, DeJong read the brief and unabashedly told the monitor what he thought was needed to get it into shape. The monitor asked DeJong if he would have time to work on it and carry out his suggestions. He responded that he did not, as he had just taken on directorship of another project and had a monograph to complete for that same monitor. A week later, DeJong's supervisor called him down to her office: "Don't you ever again tell a client that you can't do something for them!" she screamed. Lesson 1—Before reviewing his supervisor's work, DeJong should have made her aware of the monitor's request and cleared it with her. Lesson 2—DeJong had overstepped his authority in talking to the monitor about his work schedule. Whether he liked it or not, that was his supervisor's job.

Another test of our capacity for civility has been working for government monitors or supervisors who were less competent or knowledgeable than many of the staff members under them. DeJong once worked on a federal contract for a project monitor who attempted a line-by-line rewrite of his entire report. From DeJong's point of view, her "contribution" altered the meaning of the report and was decidedly unhelpful. His anger was fueled by the fact that the monitor had only a B.A. in psychology. Restrained by his supervisor from directly confronting the project monitor, DeJong endured 11 months of endless redrafting before the monitor was satisfied.

In a similar case, friction developed between Saxe and a project manager about the scope of the research work being undertaken. Saxe's reactions ran the gamut from brooding to complaining to fellow workers about the project leader's deficiencies. Finally, in a meeting he initiated with the project leader, Saxe described how hard it was for him not to have control of the research agenda. In turn, the project leader admitted that she felt threatened by Saxe's academic credentials and disliked his personal demeanor. Their clash was never fully resolved, but their discussion prevented the research project from foundering.

Because of the highly politicized environment in which much nonacademic research is funded, defined, and acted on, success in nonacademic settings requires an ability and a willingness to nurture and then use professional contacts. Quite simply, establishing links with sponsors, policymakers, and other researchers is an important part of the research business. During Saxe's year in Washington, D.C., while he worked for the Congressional Office of Technology Assessment, he became part of a group that met every other week for dinner and discussion with a political notable. Deliberately, Saxe used those dinners to establish professional contacts that could help him with his current work and perhaps bring other work his way later on. To some, that stratagem may seem like a crass exercise in Machiavellianism. Perhaps, but there is a less pejorative term for the same activity—"networking." (We hasten to add that academics do their share of networking, too, principally at professional meetings and conferences.)

Organizational survival skills. Researchers who work in nonacademic settings are ahead of the game if they have the know-how for coping with the exigencies of a large, business-oriented organization. Neither of us feels particularly savvy as organizational survivors. Between us, we have worked for many research organizations, but have survived only by keeping options open. We look with awe at those who do survive and, indeed, flourish within large bureaucracies and companies—they obtain the resources they seek, are well-compensated, and manage to survive despite frequent organizational upheavals and changes in funding priorities. Having observed the "true survivors," we can offer the following suggestions.

It is common for academics to regard their university or college as an irritant. Some half-jokingly assert, for example, that, were it not for the demands of the university—the teaching load, the office hours, the interminable faculty meetings, the paperwork—they could be truly productive. Although such cynicism is not universal, it is clear that organizational responsibilities are usually taken more lightly by academics than by others. Above all else, in a nonacademic research organization, researchers must take that organization seriously. In many academic settings, faculty can "get away" with failing to respond to memos, appearing at meetings late, or taking relatively little responsibility for others' work, but such behavior is not tolerated in nonacademic organizations.

It is also clear that nonacademic researchers must be flexible. Nonacademic research staff may be called on frequently to switch substantive areas, co-workers, or even offices. Inflexibility or even mere irritability in the face of such changes reduces a researcher's value to the organization.

DeJong once witnessed a pointed lesson on the need for flexibility when his former colleagues at Abt were put "under the gun" by a demanding research sponsor. Several research studies were underway at Abt when the funder's newly appointed director came aboard, but one project in particular captured his attention—a large-scale study of neighborhood crime prevention programs. After the television program, "Good Morning, America," announced plans to do a week-long series of news stories on crime prevention, the director ordered that the final report be ready for release that same week. This gave the researchers approximately four weeks to complete their first draft, receive comments from a panel of outside experts, and revise. Obviously, their other research work had to be put on hold. As DeJong's colleagues girded themselves for battle and bade temporary farewell to their families, rumors spread that the agency's new director hoped that the report would get him on TV. The report was completed on time, but sadly, the new director was not asked to be on "Good Morning, America."

Professional Skills

We do not mean to create the impression that success in applied research organizations depends only on researchers' social attractiveness or their ability to meet others' demands, for this simply is not the case. In fact, professional and intellectual skills are often called upon in nonacademic settings in more strenuous ways than they are in academia. In this section, we discuss three types of skills that students must develop when considering a nonacademic research career: effective oral and written communication, management skills, and intellectual breadth and adaptability.

Communication. The ability to write, speak, and communicate ideas is critical to working effectively in applied research settings. Possibly because so many other skills are required, communication skills are not normally cited as the key to a successful nonacademic research career. Yet, whether researchers are developing an internal memorandum, a funding proposal, or a final report, those skills are essential. Indeed, while "publish or perish" may be a well-known shibboleth of academia, good communication skills, especially the ability to write well, may be even more important in nonacademic settings.

Two features of good written communication are primary. The first is speed. Writing quickly is, perhaps, an art unto itself, but it is also an ability that can be developed with practice. Saxe estimates that he has improved his ability to write quickly by a factor of ten since he was in graduate school. Making a deliberate effort to quicken his writing speed, he first used dictation, then learned to compose at typewriters, and now uses word processors for almost all of his writing. The second feature of good written communication is being able to obtain and incorporate feedback. Because work is done in teams, and because supervisors often review all work, such feedback is provided routinely in most nonacademic research organizations. But receiving criticism with aplomb and then using that criticism to maximal advantage, requires a real commitment of time and effort.

Good speaking ability is another critical skill. Like their academic counterparts, nonacademic researchers need to be able to speak to both small and large groups—to hold their attention, to communicate ideas clearly, and to provide opportunities for comment and discussion. Outside the university, however, there is rarely the luxury (or, perhaps, the agony) of the one-hour lecture or three-hour seminar. Nonacademic researchers must learn to speak concisely and with the needs of the particular audience—researchers, policymakers, or both—clearly in mind.

A specialized form of public speaking is giving expert testimony before a court or a legislative committee. Saxe has given legislative testimony on a number of occasions. Each time, he has agonized over whether his oral testimony should be read directly from a shortened version of his prepared written statement or delivered extemporaneously from an outline. Once, when he read from his prepared statement, he ran over time and the Senator chairing the committee cut him off mid-sentence. On another occasion, where he talked from an outline, he later learned when reviewing a hearing transcript that he had not explained one of two key points.

Another communication skill involves dealing with the mass media. Nonacademic researchers are often involved in projects that are of great public interest. Although researchers who seek out publicity are a minority, all of them must be prepared to deal with requests for information about their research. In dealing with the press, researchers have to be more careful than usual about what they say; they must remain cognizant that the information will be summarized and rewritten without their approval, that statements can be misinterpreted, and that the media can make even insignificant points "larger than life." But it is also important for researchers to recognize that a relationship with the media can be controlled—they have the right to check whether a reporter has correctly understood what has been said and to know exactly what will be done with the information provided.

Management skills. The second set of professional skills necessary for effective work in nonacademic research is management skills. Nonacademic researchers must learn to manage their time and their relationships with subordinates and to negotiate with research sponsors, fellow team members, and supervisors.

Although the contrast with academia may be overstated, timeliness and smooth teamwork are given far more serious consideration in nonacademic settings. At the university, academics are their own boss. Beyond showing up for classes and getting grades in on time, they have few scheduled demands on their time. In nonacademic organizations, it is far different. Because researchers are dependent on one another for completing their work, each researchers timeliness is essential. Everything—proposals, budgets, staffing plans, final reports—has deadlines, and researchers are expected to meet them.

Almost all of the work Saxe has done for the Congressional Office of Technology Assessment (OTA) has been completed under severe time constraints. For example, in a study he conducted for OTA on the validity of polygraph test (see Saxe, Dougherty, & Cross, 1985), approximately six months were available to conduct the study. Controversy over polygraph testing has existed for 70 years, but as a result of a presidential order that would have expanded government use of such tests, Congress needed to review the issue within its current session. The ability of Saxe and his co-workers to conduct the study within the alloted time was as critical to their success as the scientific validity of their conclusions.

Whereas academics usually have an ambiguous managerial role, such responsibilities are apt to be more formal in nonacademic settings. Perhaps because of our academic ties, and because of our sensitivity to how we have been supervised in the past, both of us are eager to guarantee that our supervision is well received; we try to ensure that each member of the team feels valued and has a voice in the shape of the project. This approach seems to work well as long as the project staff are competent and hardworking. But when they are not? Termination of employment is not always an option when higher-echelon supervisors assign staff to projects and project managers are expected to make the best of it. Our principal advice to those who have yet to venture outside academia is to be aware that personnel issues can consume an inordinate amount of time and energy.

A final management issue has to do with the ability to negotiate. Schedules, while often fixed, are often negotiable, as are budgets, work requirements, and even the definition of a research approach. Nonacademic researchers have to learn how to work with others toward the resolution of problems that invariably develop because of constraints imposed by research sponsors or organizations, by the needs and abilities of staff members, and by conflicting demands from supervisors. Not only do researchers have to learn to compromise, but they have to learn to express themselves directly and to listen to others' points of view. While academics are rewarded for fighting for their ideas, come what may, researchers in nonacademic settings cannot afford to regard every decision about a research project as a "win/lose" competition. To do so is ultimately self-defeating.

A common area of difficulty in applied research studies is negotiation of the research design with program sponsors. Researchers often feel caught between their concerns for the validity of their design and the concerns—logistical, political, or ethical—of research funders. To the extent that researchers regard the sponsors' concerns as extraneous to the more important objective of establishing research validity, satisfactory negotiations will be impossible. Nonacademic researchers must learn that a research design has to be adapted to the overall research context. Compromises have to be made.

Intellectual breadth and adaptability. Up to this point, we have said little about the need for nonacademic researchers to have sharp methodological and analytical skills. Obviously, such skills are critical. In this respect, there is no difference between academic and nonacademic research settings. It is our contention, however, that applied research requires a greater flexibility in approach (see Kahle, 1983). In basic research, a researcher can "mine" an idea using a single methodology for a long period of time. That is rarely the case in applied research. Typically, each applied problem requires a different set of methods. Campbell (1971) has characterized the role of applied researchers as "methodological servants": in applied research, others may define the problem area, but researchers have responsibility for devising the means of studying it.

To prepare for such work, nonacademic researchers must be familiar with a wide range of methodological approaches—e.g., qualitative case study analysis, ethnographic observation, focus group interviews. And such work often requires greater statistical sophistication as well. Analysis of variance, usually involving two-or three-factor experiments, has characterized much of psychological research over the past 20 years, and ANOVA procedures are usually at the center of methodological training for psychology graduate students. Yet, those not familiar with other multivariate techniques will be at a loss when problems require causal modeling and other analytic solutions. Nonacademic researchers have to know what other statistical techniques are available and be flexible enough to consider them as solutions. Of course, such statistical sophistication may not always be useful. Analyses that cannot be explained or understood easily by policymakers should also be avoided.

Nonacademic researchers need to be conceptually flexible as well. Much of traditional graduate training in psychology amounts to a socialization process, during which students learn particular paradigms. But such paradigms may not be appropriate for certain research problems encountered in nonacademic work. Researchers thrust into interdisciplinary settings must be open enough to learn about other perspectives, to appreciate what they have to offer, and when appropriate, to incorporate them. We are not suggesting that psychologists be "intellectual chameleons" for the sake of doing nonacademic research. Quite to the contrary, we believe that psychologists bring both a unique theoretical perspective that should be heard and a methodological rigor and discipline that enable them to contribute significantly to applied research.

CONCLUDING COMMENTS

Both of us were trained in traditional social psychology programs. Our background in laboratory research—involving clean designs, yet often nongeneralizable findings—did not fully prepare us to do work of interest to government and corporate policymakers. Our sheltered life in the academy did not fully prepare us for work settings in which others define the research agenda and a wholly different set of norms operates. We made the plunge into nonacademic research work anyway. Despite the mistakes we made along the way as we developed the interpersonal and intellectual skills that such work requires, we are both glad to be doing the work we do.

We said in our introduction that we hoped to encourage new psychologists to travel beyond their present boundaries and to consider doing applied work in nonacademic settings. Obviously, by enumerating the frustration we have encountered there, we have not described a Shangri-La—the scenery is beautiful, and the natives are mostly a friendly lot, but there are pickpockets about, and the fresh vegetables are sometimes suspect. We thought you should know that in advance. But also believe that these detractions are not so great that others should be afraid to join us. We hope that this brief chapter has helped new psychologists better understand the demands of nonacademic research settings and that they will therefore better enjoy the rewards that applied work can bring.

ACKNOWLEDGMENTS

There are several people we want to thank whose ideas and experiences helped us in preparing this chapter: Anne-Marie Baronas, Michelle Fine, Ronald W. Geddes, Gail A. Goolkasian, Robert Kraut, Joan Petersilia, Michael J. Saks, Bradford Smith, and Susan Solomon.

REFERENCES

Campbell, D. T. (August, 1971). *Methods for the experimenting society.* Paper presented at the meetings of the American Psychological Association, Washington, DC.

Hershoff, L. F. (1956). *The compleat cruiser: The art, practice, and enjoyment of boating.* White Plains, NY: Sheridan House.

Kahle, L. R. (1983). Two needed trends in training social psychologists. *SASP Newsletter, 9*(5), 6–7.

Pion, G. M., & Lipsey, M. W. (1984). Psychology and society: The challenge of change. *American Psychologist, 39,* 739–754.

Rosenblum, R., & McGillis, D. (1979). Observations on the role of consultants in the public sector. *Public Administration Review, 39,* 219–226.

Saxe, L. (1983). The perspective of social psychology: Toward a viable model for application. In R. F. Kidd & M. J. Saks (Eds.), *Advances in applied social psychology,* Vol. 2, Hillsdale, NJ: Lawrence Erlbaum Associates.

Saxe, L., & Dougherty, D. (1985). Technology assessment and Congressional use of social psychology: Making complexity useful. In S. Oskamp (Ed.), *Applied social psychology annual* (Vol. 6). Beverly Hills, CA: Sage.

Saxe, L., Dougherty, D., & Cross, T. (1985). The validity of polygraph testing. *American Psychologist, 40,* 355–366.

Walton, I. (1931). *The compleat angler: Or, the contemplative man's recreation.* Philadelphia: McKay. (original work published in 1653)

Weiss, C. H. (1977). Research for policy's sake: The enlightenment function of social research. *Policy Analysis, 4,* 531–543.

Wholey, J. S. (1979). *Evaluation: Promise and performance.* Washington, DC: Urban Institute.

---

[1]Policymakers do not always act on research findings, however. Weiss (1977) has noted that "government decisionmakers tend to use research indirectly, as a source of ideas, information and orientations to the world" (p. 531). She outlines two principal reasons for this: (1) policymakers are pressed by demands that conflict with the recommendations emerging from research; and (2) policymakers sometimes fail to define their research needs adequately (see also Wholey, 1979).

---

[2]The discussion that follows is based primarily on the perspective of researchers working in nonacademic settings on projects supported by their organization or by an external funding agency. Although many psychologists work as funders of such projects in their role as government or foundation staff, the more frequent experience of being a grant or contract recipient is emphasized here.

APPENDIX: RECOMMENDED READINGS

1. Aronson, Elliot (1977). Research in social psychology as a leap of faith. *Personality and Social Psychology Bulletin, 3,* 190–195.

   In this article Aronson presents his philosophy of how to do research in social psychology. This article will be of interest to anyone who has ever wondered what to do research on as well as those of us who have had occasion to conduct a less than perfect experiment.

2. Gleitman, Henry (1984). Introducing psychology. *American Psychologist, 39,* 421–427.

   In this article Gleitman presents his views about teaching introductory psychology. This article will not only be of interest to those who teach this course, but also to those committed to providing a liberal arts education to undergraduate students in whatever course they teach.